The Folk Remedy Encyclopedia

Olive Oil, Vinegar, Honey and 1,001 other Home Remedies

By the Editors of FC&A Medical Publishing

Publisher's Note

The editors of FC&A have taken careful measures to ensure the accuracy and usefulness of the information in this book. While every attempt has been made to assure accuracy, errors may occur. We advise readers to carefully review and understand the ideas and tips presented and to seek the advice of a qualified professional before attempting to use them. The publisher and editors disclaim all liability (including any injuries, damages or losses) resulting from the use of the information in this book.

The health information in this book is for information only and is not intended to be a medical guide for self-treatment. It does not constitute medical advice and should not be construed as such or used in place of your doctor's medical advice.

Therefore we do not lose heart. Though outwardly we are wasting away, yet inwardly we are being renewed day by day. For our light and momentary troubles are achieving for us an eternal glory that far outweighs them all. So we fix our eyes not on what is seen, but on what is unseen. For what is seen is temporary, but what is unseen is eternal.

2 Corinthians 4:16-18

FC&A
103 Clover Green
Peachtree City, GA 30269

Produced by the staff of FC&A

First printing December 2001

ISBN 1-890957-57-7 HC

CONTENTS

Diabetes .90

Diarrhea 108

Eyestrain 114

Food poisoning 120

Gingivitis 132

Headaches 137

Insomnia 204

Irritable bowel syndrome 212

Kidney stones 217

Lactose intolerance 222

Memory loss 225

Menopause 230

Muscle pain 238

FOLK REMEDY SECRETS

Explore the world of home remedies

Long ago, you might have treated a toothache by cutting a wart off a horse's leg and rubbing it on your gums. Or you might have smeared fresh cow dung on your chest to chase away a cold.

While neither of those old-time folk remedies seems very appealing — or effective — there are plenty of home remedies that do work. We've tracked them down and collected them for you in this amazing book.

Let *The Folk Remedy Encyclopedia: Olive Oil, Vinegar, Honey and 1,001 Other Home Remedies* be your guide to sensible, do-it-yourself treatments. You'll read about herbal remedies, ancient healing secrets, and other natural ways to fight illness. You'll also hear from modern health experts and get a glimpse into the latest medical research.

It might surprise you how often science proves what Granny knew all along — you don't always have to shell out a fortune for doctor's visits, prescription drugs, or surgery. Often, you can treat your condition with items from your own kitchen. Olive oil, vinegar, and honey, just to name a few, work wonders for dozens of ailments.

1

For your convenience, we've organized *The Folk Remedy Encyclopedia* alphabetically by condition, from "Allergy" to "Wrinkles." Each section includes a handy box that briefly explains the condition and its symptoms. Go straight to the condition that interests you, or just browse through the book for exciting, useful information. Keep your eyes open for helpful and fun "Folk Remedy" tidbits scattered throughout the book, too.

Read on to explore the wonderful world of home remedies. We hope you'll enjoy these fascinating treatments that will help restore your health and improve your quality of life.

The Editors of FC&A

ALLERGY

Food allergies: Take back control of your life

Do you suffer from a true food allergy or merely a food sensitivity? The answer could mean life or death.

It's easy to confuse the two conditions, warns Dr. Hugh A. Sampson, Chief of the Jaffe Food Allergy Institute at the Mount Sinai School of Medicine in New York, since they can have many of the same symptoms. But while a food intolerance can be an uncomfortable annoyance, a food allergy can turn into a deadly reaction.

According to Sampson, "An intolerance is a non-immunologic response." This means your body's reaction has nothing to do with your immune system. You suffer from lactose intolerance, for example, if your digestive system doesn't make enough lactase, an enzyme that breaks down the sugar in dairy foods. Other substances that cause different reactions include sulfites, histamines, monosodium glutamate (MSG), red wine, chocolate, and artificial food colors.

What is it?

You are considered allergic if your immune system over-responds to a usually harmless substance. Called allergens, these substances can range from pollen to peanuts to poison ivy. Your eyes, respiratory system, digestive system, and skin are most often affected. Allergic reactions, which run in families, can range from a few sneezes to life-threatening anaphylactic shock.

Symptoms:
- Skin rash or hives
- Stuffy nose, sneezing
- Coughing, difficulty breathing
- Red, watery eyes
- Stomach cramps, bloating, diarrhea, or vomiting

3

A true food allergy, though, is your immune system overreacting to certain foods. "With a food allergy," Sampson explains, "other organs come in." For example, your skin might break out in a rash, your mouth might tingle, or your throat might tighten up, causing coughing, wheezing, and choking. The worse case scenario — anaphylactic shock — causes your blood pressure to drop dangerously low and your windpipe to close up. Every year, allergic food reactions hit 30,000 people, killing 150 of them.

According to Sampson, although food allergies mostly occur during childhood, some carry over into adulthood. Occasionally, they suddenly appear in adults who never had a problem before.

Hundreds of foods can cause a reaction, but the Big Eight are shellfish; peanuts; tree nuts like walnuts, cashews, pecans, and almonds; milk; eggs; fish; soybeans; and wheat. Recently, experts discovered that even such an unlikely food as zucchini can bring on a reaction. So can inulin, a carbohydrate found in some processed foods and in vegetables like artichokes and chicory.

As dangerous as food allergies are, you can learn to manage them safely.

Get a diagnosis. When you have a reaction after eating a food, notify your doctor immediately. She can determine and begin treating the real cause, whether it's an allergy, an intolerance, or something totally different like a case of food poisoning, celiac disease, or an ulcer. She may even refer you to an allergist.

And remember to tell a new doctor about your allergies. She'll need to know in order to give you proper treatment and care.

Keep a diary. An accurate record of what and when you eat can help your doctor pinpoint exactly what's ailing you. Also, note your symptoms, how the food was prepared, and if anyone else got sick.

Learn your trouble foods. Ask your doctor about cross-sensitization. This means you could be allergic to a "family" of foods — a reaction to shrimp could be a sign of an allergy to lobster or crab as well.

On the other hand, oils made from certain foods, like peanuts or soybeans, are often safe to eat since the refining process removes most of the allergy-causing ingredients. However, there are always exceptions, including cold-pressed and foreign-processed oils and those used in restaurants. Talk with your doctor before trying different oils.

Ask the chef. Eating at restaurants can be the trickiest feat facing an allergy victim. The two biggest dangers are hidden ingredients in sauces, dressings, etc. and cross-contamination — when allergens get into foods unexpectedly.

A chef, for instance, could use the same spoon in your veggie stir-fry that he used in his peanut chicken. If you're very sensitive to nuts, that would be enough to cause a deadly reaction.

Prevent this from happening by asking questions. Double-check ingredients listed in the menu, and don't hesitate to quiz your waiter or even the chef about the exact ingredients of a dish. If they think you're nutty, remind them you could die from eating the wrong food. In fact, they'll take your questions more seriously if you let them know you're allergic.

Be wary of ingredient lists. Packaged foods can hide your allergen where you least expect it. Snack cakes, for instance, can contain small amounts of nuts, and that soup packet might be enriched with powdered milk. Labels don't always say when products contain one of the Big Eight. Recently, the Food Allergy Issues Alliance suggested the food industry begin simply and clearly labeling products containing major food allergens. The FDA also plans to get involved, promising to spot-check food-processing plants to make sure allergy-causing foods are not contaminating other foods by accident.

Just say no. Doctors do not have a cure for food allergies yet, so sometimes it's safest just to avoid a type of food or restaurant altogether, says Sampson. Chinese restaurants could be one no-no for peanut allergy sufferers since the chance of cross-contamination is high. Restaurant desserts often contain flavorings or extracts that even the chef won't know about. And street vendors might be less likely to reveal allergy-causing ingredients.

Wash away allergens. Good kitchen hygiene is a big part of guarding against cross-contamination, says the Food Allergy and Anaphylaxis Network. After using any utensil, cutting board, pot, or pan, it's important to wash it carefully with soap and hot water to remove all allergen particles.

Carry emergency medication. Sampson says wherever you go, medicine to stop allergic reactions should go, too. The most common emergency treatment — a shot of epinephrine or adrenaline — requires a prescription. That's one more reason to see a doctor about your condition.

Wear medical alert info. In case you suffer anaphylactic shock, emergency medical personnel need to know exactly what is wrong and what needs to be done.

Have a positive attitude. Just because you have a food allergy doesn't mean you have to live on bread and water. You can still eat many of the foods you enjoy. If you need support from other allergy sufferers, not to mention advice from medical experts, Sampson suggests contacting the Food Allergy and Anaphylaxis Network. Either visit them at their Web site at <www.foodallergy.org> or contact them the old-fashioned way at:

> 10400 Eaton Place
> Suite 107
> Fairfax, VA 22030-2208
> 800-929-4040

Discover hidden sources of skin rash

You use them to stay healthy and beautiful, but the toiletries you rely on every day might be your skin's worst enemy. Perfumes, moisturizers, sunscreens, astringents, deodorants, antiperspirants, shampoos, soaps, dyes, and nail polishes — the average adult uses at least seven of these skin care products every day. These, plus toilet paper, tissues, dryer sheets, and household cleaning products, all contain ingredients that could irritate your skin.

To become more aware of hidden chemicals, read product labels for known rash offenders, like fragrances, preservatives, and the skin conditioner lanolin. But even with this precaution, you still might not learn all the ingredients, since companies don't always accurately report every additive in their products. In fact, a recent study of 67 different skin creams found that almost half of them were mislabeled.

Here's how to save your skin from potential troublemakers.

Ration the soap and water. Healthy skin is your first line of defense against allergic reactions and infection. Dried and cracked skin allows bacteria a direct route to your bloodstream. If your skin's already dry, choose only mild soaps (like beauty bars) or soap-free cleansers. Use as little as possible, lather with lukewarm water, and rinse with cool water. After a shower or bath, rub in a moisturizer to fight future dryness.

Nurture your nails. According to the American Academy of Dermatology (AAD), allergic reactions are the most common problem caused by nail-care products. You can develop itching, burning, and pain under or around your nail and even on your face and neck. Acrylic nails, polish, and nail hardeners contain formaldehyde and other compounds that often cause reactions. If you go to a salon for artificial nails, make sure they don't use methacrylate (MMA), a product banned in many states. The AAD says to notice very strong odors in the salon, extremely hard artificial nails, or ones that don't soak off easily. These signs of MMA call for a report to your state board of health.

Appraise your jewelry. If you develop a rash after wearing a piece of jewelry, you are probably allergic to the nickel in it. Try stainless steel or other nickel-free jewelry instead. Even if you're not allergic to your jewelry, take it all off when you wash. Rings and other pieces can trap rash-causing wetness near your skin.

Forget the fragrance. Whether it's shampoo, hairspray, or body lotion, most items in your bathroom contain fragrances. Even products labeled "unscented" include something to mask the unpleasant smells of their chemicals. If you need to be sure about hidden fragrances, look for "fragrance-free" or "without perfume" on the package.

Mind your makeup. Stick with hypoallergenic, noncomedogenic, and nonacnegenic brands. They're the healthiest for your skin because they cause fewer allergies and won't clog your pores. It's also a good idea to use water-soluble cosmetics, since you won't need harsh solvents to remove them. Replace eye makeup every three months and never share cosmetics.

Beware of hair care. Always test hair color first on a patch of skin, like behind your ear or the inside of your elbow. When it comes to curls, give your hair a break. Wait at least three months between perms and ask your hairdresser about gentle, non-irritating products.

Avoid antiperspirant allergies. Don't use your deodorant on irritated skin or just-shaved areas. And be careful not to apply them outside your armpits — this skin can be more sensitive.

Reconsider rubber. Experts say to wear gloves when you're working around the house or in the garden. They can protect your hands from harsh chemicals, drying cleansers, and allergy-causing plants. Be careful, though — you might be allergic to the rubber found in some gloves. You'll know by the itching and burning you'll feel wherever the rubber touches your skin. You could even develop hives. Rubber elastic bands in clothing can bring on this reaction in some people, too. If this is the case for you, don't give up on gloves and underwear. Just switch to products made of some other material, like cloth, vinyl, or leather.

In most cases, you don't need to be Sherlock Holmes to figure out what is causing your rash. Test your theory by avoiding the product to see if your rash goes away. If you still aren't sure, give up all of your skin care products at the same time.

No matter what causes your skin condition, make sure to visit your dermatologist any time you have a severe reaction.

Simple solutions that will scratch your itch

It's easy to irritate your skin. Anything from the sun to toxic plants, dust mites, and other pests can cause allergic rashes, itching, and sores. But now it's easy — and cheap — to treat these kinds of reactions. Just don't rush out and pay a fortune for expensive creams and ointments. Try some natural remedies that won't rub your sensitive skin the wrong way.

Brew a healing pot. Just a few cups of oolong tea may let you say so long to itchy, scaly skin caused by a type of allergic disorder called dermatitis. In a clinical trial, drinking one liter of this Chinese beverage every day improved symptoms within one or two weeks. At the end of a month, two-thirds of those in the study reported relief. Experts believe oolong tea contains certain compounds that block allergic reactions.

Resurrect an ancient cure. Aloe vera may have been one of the key ingredients used to preserve ancient Egyptian mummies. But you don't have to wait hundreds of years for its skin-saving benefits.

The soothing liquid found inside the plump leaves of the aloe vera plant relieves all kinds of skin problems. Use it fresh or substitute one of the many aloe-based products you'll find at the drugstore.

Aloe creams, gels, and lotions soothe itches, rashes, sunburn, and blisters. Apply aloe lip balm to ease painful cold sores, and drink aloe juice for mouth ulcers. Remember though, these products vary in quality and strength. If you don't get results with one, try a different brand or go to the more dependable living plant.

Doctor it with dairy. The uncomfortable itching of poison oak or ivy can ruin the fun of a day outdoors, but you may find relief inside your refrigerator. Make a soothing milk compress by soaking a clean cloth — linen, gauze, and soft flannel are good choices — in cool whole milk. Place it loosely on the affected area for 10 to 20 minutes every hour until your skin feels better. This works well with painful sunburn and other skin conditions, too.

Gather a bouquet of healing blooms. Pick pot or garden marigolds, also known as calendula, for a colorful posy or a tea to soothe irritated skin. Steep the flowers in water and place a tea-soaked cloth over your rash. You'll be amazed at how much better you'll feel. In addition, use the calendula tea as a rinse for sores in your mouth. Calendula also comes in oils, creams, and ointments that help wounds heal fast.

Another flower, chamomile, contains its own healing ingredient. In European tests, chamomile cream was almost as effective as hydrocortisone in relieving some skin problems.

Apply a poultice. You may not know what a poultice is, but if you're suffering from a skin rash, you'll want to try one right away. This old-fashioned remedy is basically any warm, thick mixture of herbs, water, and other ingredients that you spread on your skin and cover with a cloth.

A witch hazel poultice can help dry up an oozing rash and relieve the pain. Stir 5 to 10 heaping teaspoons of finely chopped witch hazel leaves into a cup of water. Bring this to a boil and simmer for five to 10 minutes, then strain. Press the wet leaves against your rash and cover the area with a warm cloth to hold it in place.

A poultice made from crushed flax seeds mixed with hot water can also soothe and protect your irritated skin.

Say "nuts" to a skin annoyance. Tannins in the leaves of the English walnut tree act as an astringent, tightening skin tissues and helping dry up any discharge. Boil 5 teaspoons chopped leaves in a cup of water. Strain this mixture and soak a soft cloth in the liquid. Apply the compress two to four times a day.

Another nutty solution to a variety of skin problems is almond oil. You'll often find it in commercial lotions and ointments that soften and soothe the skin. Experts consider almond oil safe, but if you have food allergies, consider a different treatment.

End eczema agony with breakthrough treatment

A fungus found at the foot of Mount Tsukuba in Japan might be the best hope yet for treating the intense itching, swelling, cracking, and inflammation of eczema.

About one out of every 17 people suffers from this chronic skin disease, also called atopic dermatitis. Although doctors often prescribe steroids for eczema, they don't always work and can have serious side effects.

It's been 40 years since eczema sufferers have seen any new treatments. That's why scientists are so excited about a new class of steroid-free medications, called topical immunomodulators (TIMs) made from the Japanese fungus. Two of these, tacrolimus and ascomycin, are showing incredible clinical success — clearing eczema in more than 80 percent of treated patients with few side effects.

If you've been living with the physical and social discomfort of eczema, talk to your dermatologist about TIMs.

Soak your troubles away. A relaxing bath may be just the thing to relieve allergic symptoms — just leave out the bubbles and turn down the heat. Instead, mix some oatmeal, baking soda, or vinegar in a tub of cool water to ease the itching. For the discomforts of poison oak or ivy, also try spreading a thick paste of baking soda and water over the affected area.

Laugh your rash off. Humor may truly be the best medicine when it comes to allergies. Japanese researchers exposed people with a history of allergic reactions to various allergens. Welts appeared, but shrank in those who watched a classic Charlie Chaplin film. Welts stayed the same in those who watched a weather report instead. Find out what tickles your funny bone — it just may save your skin.

Breathe easy without hay fever misery

Play it smart and you can survive any attack of pollen, mold, or other source of seasonal allergy. Sneezing, sniffling, headaches, itchy eyes — these symptoms of "hay fever" can make you dread the approach of spring and summer. But follow these tips from the American Academy of Allergy, Asthma and Immunology and breathe new life into allergy season.

Work out inside. If you walk for exercise, try hotfooting it around the inside of a shopping mall. It's cool, safe, and a great social activity, too. If you must be outside, avoid grassy or wooded areas.

Close those windows. You may never see it, but your nose will certainly feel that pollen and mold blowing into your house or car. During allergy season, keep windows shut at home and when driving.

Improve your air. Use an air conditioner and dehumidifier to keep your home cool and dry. Not only will you filter out pollen and mold, but you'll also get rid of dust mites, another source of allergies.

Keep your house at less than 51 percent humidity, and you could have 10 times fewer allergens. Simply walking into a home with a dehumidifier may help you breathe easier within minutes.

Keep an eye on the numbers. Pay attention to pollen counts in your area, and stay inside when they're high. To find your local pollen count online, visit the National Allergy Bureau at <www.aaaai.org/nab>.

Avoid yard work. Don't stir up mold and pollen by mowing or raking your grass. If you can't hire the job out for a few months, at least wear a paper mask.

Use a dryer. Don't hang laundry on an outside clothesline where it can pick up pollen and mold spores.

Be a sneeze-free friend

Flowers may not always be the thoughtful gift you intend them to be. Even if you don't suffer from allergies, others might. In a recent survey, one out of eight people admitted to a hospital developed rhinitis, an allergic reaction that causes a stuffy nose. The culprit — those lovely bouquets from well-meaning friends and relatives. So, the next time you're looking to perk someone up, choose crossword puzzles, a book, video, or fruit. Just leave the pollen outside.

Flowers aren't the only guilty party, either. Pet owners should know, even if you leave Kitty at home, his allergens will more than likely hitch a ride. You can carry around enough cat dander on your clothes to cause a reaction in allergic co-workers or neighbors. Fuzzy, fluffy, or wooly clothes are magnets for cat dander, while freshly washed clothes will cause the least sneezing and sniffling.

Lather up. Shower and wash your hair after being outdoors. Allergens can cling to you, bringing hay fever misery inside.

If you follow these tips and still suffer, don't despair. Scientists have developed a new class of drugs that work on your eyes and nose — the receptor sites for allergens, says Zab Mohsenifar M.D., director of the Division of Pulmonary/Critical Care medicine at Cedars-Sinai Medical Center.

Called anti-immunoglobulin E (anti-IgE) drugs, they not only fight allergy symptoms, but they do it without making you sleepy like most allergy medicines. "These new medications," says Mohsenifar, "train the cells at the receptors' sites so they do not recognize allergens as foreign bodies. Thus, there is no vigorous reaction, and the chain reaction is stopped at a very early stage."

Although scientists are still testing anti-IgE drugs, Mohsenifar thinks they will soon be widely used. That's good news for anyone who wants to give hay fever a breather.

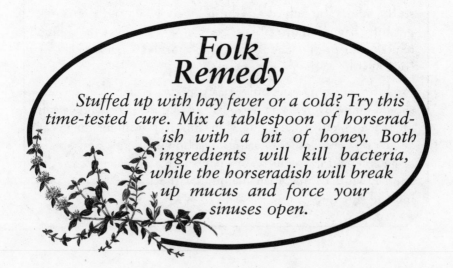

Folk
Remedy

Stuffed up with hay fever or a cold? Try this time-tested cure. Mix a tablespoon of horseradish with a bit of honey. Both ingredients will kill bacteria, while the horseradish will break up mucus and force your sinuses open.

ALZHEIMER'S DISEASE

Secret to cutting your Alzheimer's risk

Want to lower your risk of Alzheimer's? Then start by cutting calories, and while you're at it, cut your couch-potato time. Research shows that a low-calorie diet combined with exercise will help keep your brain young and may even shield you from this memory-robbing disease.

According to experts, the secret is simple — use your head when it comes to how you live. Make a few sensible and healthy changes in your lifestyle today, starting with your diet.

Cut extra calories. The key to keeping your brain in top form may be a low-calorie diet. The older you get, the more your brain cells are damaged by inflammation and oxidation, two major risk factors for Alzheimer's. The cells also have a harder time repairing themselves.

What is it?

Dementia is any loss of mental ability that is severe enough to interfere with your everyday life. Alzheimer's disease is the most common type of dementia in older people.

With this mental disorder, brain cells gradually die, and you generate fewer chemical signals that help you function. Over time, memory, thinking, and behavior deteriorate. There is no known cause or cure.

Symptoms:
- Increasing forgetfulness
- Language difficulties
- Anxiety
- Personality changes
- Depression
- Difficulty making decisions

But a study of mice showed that a low-calorie diet might have a great effect on brain aging. When scientists compared the brain cells of "senior" mice fed a low-calorie diet to those of similar mice on a traditional diet, they found a remarkable difference. The brain cells of the low-cal mice continued to function as if they were younger.

Trim the fat. While you're cutting calories, also keep an eye on the amount of fat you eat. Studies show your risk of developing Alzheimer's is more than seven times higher if you eat a high-fat diet. Although this relationship only seems true for people with the "Alzheimer's gene" — called Apolipoprotein E4 — you can never lose by eating a heart-healthy, low-fat diet.

"A diet high in antioxidants — fruits and veggies — and low in fat and meat, high in fish is protective against the disease," affirms Dr. Robert P. Friedland, one of the researchers on the study.

Load up on nutrients. More than any other organ in your body, your brain needs a daily supply of hi-test fuel — a mixture of all the essential nutrients.

- **B vitamins.** "I recommend that people take B vitamins," Friedland says, "which will lower their plasma homocysteine level, which is a risk factor for [Alzheimer's] as well as stroke and heart disease." Friedland is mindful of recent research that showed people deficient in these vitamins have poorer thinking and memory skills. Other studies suggest a diet supplemented with B vitamins might actually improve your brainpower. Eating fruits, vegetables, whole grains, dairy, and lean meats will give you a brain-boosting supply of folate, thiamin, and other B vitamins.

- **Antioxidants.** Free radicals are unstable chemicals that cause damage linked to cancer, heart disease — and now memory loss and Alzheimer's. Antioxidants, which prevent and repair this damage, might lower your risk of developing Alzheimer's by almost 25 per-cent, according to a recent European study. For an antioxidant-rich diet, eat a variety of vegetables as well as foods containing vitamins C and E.

◆ **Calcium.** Calcium already appears to fight breast and colon cancer, defeat digestion problems, help high blood pressure, and shore up fragile bones. Now add to that list prevent memory loss, senility, and forms of dementia like Alzheimer's. Calcium, experts say, plays a role in the way brain and nerve cells work together. So, don't fall short. Include low-fat dairy products in your diet, take your orange juice fortified with calcium, and remember to eat beans and broccoli. If you're still concerned, talk with your doctor about supplements.

Sugar may sweeten your memory

According to Mary Poppins, a spoonful of sugar helps the medicine go down. But research shows it may do even more — it may help you remember to take your medicine.

In one study, participants fasted overnight. Then, in the morning, they drank lemonade that had been sweetened either with sugar or a sugar substitute. Those who got the lemonade with sugar performed much better at a memory test than those who got the artificial sweetener.

Treating yourself to a sweet snack each day won't hurt as long as you don't go overboard. And it may even give your brain the little boost it needs to remember where you left your keys.

Escape the menace of Alzheimer's

The calorie count of a diet soda is pretty attractive if you're watching your weight — it's zero. But the artificial sweetener that saves you all those calories may harm your brain in the long run. A new study has found that aspartame, the artificial sweetener in most diet drinks, may cause memory loss.

Students at Texas Christian University who regularly drank diet sodas with aspartame were more likely than those who didn't use aspartame to experience long-term memory problems, researchers found. While they did just as well as non-users in laboratory memory tests, they were more likely to forget details of personal routines or whether they had completed a task.

This doesn't mean you have to ditch your diet drinks completely. Other studies on the effects of aspartame have had mixed results. But if you want to play it safe, perhaps you should switch to another no-calorie beverage — water. And while you're at it, follow these other simple steps to protect your memory and help keep Alzheimer's at bay.

Control blood pressure and cholesterol. New evidence shows high blood pressure and high cholesterol not only damage your heart, they may also harm your brain. So it's more important than ever to control those conditions by exercising, eating right, and getting regular check ups.

If you can't control your cholesterol and blood pressure naturally, you may have to take medication. Luckily, some heart-protecting drugs may also protect against Alzheimer's, giving you a double dose of defense. A recent study at Boston University School of Medicine found statin cholesterol medicines lowered risk of dementia by up to 70 percent. Another study found two particular types of statins — lovastatin and pravastatin — protected against AD, but a third — simvastatin — did not. Other types of cholesterol medicines also did not lower the risk of Alzheimer's, so if you're interested in this potential treatment, you need to discuss your medication with your doctor.

Reach for some aspirin. Doctors often recommend aspirin to help prevent heart disease. Now research finds regular use of aspirin may also help you avoid Alzheimer's. Other nonsteroidal anti-inflammatory drugs (NSAIDs) may put the brakes on this disease as well. One study found the popular pain-reliever ibuprofen lowered the risk of AD by 60 percent. These inexpensive remedies may be just what you need to stem the tide of Alzheimer's, but they can have serious side effects like stomach irritation and bleeding. Talk to your doctor before starting any treatment.

Consider the benefits of estrogen. Estrogen replacement therapy (ERT) may do more than ease hot flashes — it could keep your mind sharper. Several studies have found ERT lowers your risk of developing Alzheimer's disease and other dementia. It may even give your memory a boost right now. A recent study found that women on ERT performed better on tests of mental abilities. The results were supported by brain images showing estrogen users had more blood flow to the hippocampus, an area of the brain involved in memory formation.

But not all research supports estrogen as a way to fend off Alzheimer's. Two recent studies found ERT did not improve the mental abilities of women who already had the disease. And another study found estrogen helped protect against Alzheimer's only in women with certain genes.

As usual, you need to look at all sides of the issue and talk to your doctor about whether ERT is right for you. But if you decide to take estrogen for other reasons, there's a chance your brain may benefit as well.

Build up your knowledge. An excellent way to protect your brain is to flex your mental muscle often. Every time you learn something, you establish new connections between brain cells, called synapses. Alzheimer's disease destroys synapses, but experts believe the more you have, the longer it takes AD to affect your mental abilities.

You don't have to go back to school to maintain your brain, either. Any kind of learning is useful, so take up a new hobby, work crossword puzzles, or read a variety of interesting books. Everything you learn builds a reserve of knowledge that may protect your brain from the ravages of Alzheimer's disease.

Make an effort to exercise. While you're building your brain, don't neglect your body. According to research, regular exercise not only improves your heart but your mind as well. A fit heart and clear arteries supply your brain with fresh, oxygen-filled blood. This, in turn, helps guard against memory loss and Alzheimer's.

In one study, a group of seniors found that four months in an exercise routine — walking, running, or riding a stationary bike for 30 minutes a day, three days a week — improved their memory and problem-solving skills. And every step counts, according to a study of almost 6,000 women ages 65 and older. Every extra mile a week the women walked reduced their risk of mental decline by 13 percent.

Find time to socialize. Have fun and stimulate your brain at the same time by going out often with friends and family. Research finds that people who engage in lots of leisure activities such as visiting with friends, doing volunteer work, and going to church are much less likely to lose their mental abilities as they grow older.

Fend off falls to protect memories

You may be more worried about breaking your hip than injuring your head in a fall. But new research shows that even a mild concussion can damage your brain as much as being in a coma. And if you suffered a head injury when you were younger, you may be more likely to get Alzheimer's — and get it sooner.

A recent study examined records of World War II veterans to see if those who had suffered head injuries as young adults were more likely to develop Alzheimer's disease. Lead researcher Dr. Brenda Plassman of Duke University Medical School believes the study supports such a link.

"Individuals with a history of a moderate head injury were twice as likely to develop Alzheimer's disease or other types of dementia," she says. "And individuals with a history of severe head injury were about four times more likely to develop Alzheimer's disease or other types of dementia."

A previous Mayo Clinic study had shown that sustaining a head injury also might make you develop Alzheimer's sooner than normal. Researchers compared people with Alzheimer's who had suffered severe head traumas to those who were injury free. They found that the trauma victims developed the disease about eight years earlier than the others.

Since no one knows exactly how Alzheimer's develops, avoiding head injuries may be one way you can help cut your risk. Preventing falls is an important step, particularly for older adults, who are more likely to take a spill. A few simple precautions can help protect your bones and your brain.

Wear sensible shoes. Fashion should take a backseat to balance when you're choosing shoes. Steer away from high heels or thick-soled shoes that may make you unstable. That includes athletic shoes, whose rubber-tipped front may catch more easily on the floor. Go with comfortable, well-fitting oxfords or regular thick-soled sneakers with laces, and keep those laces tied.

Check your medications. Some medicines can make you dizzy as a side effect, which could increase your risk of falling. Whenever your doctor prescribes a new medicine, ask him about potential side effects. If you find your prescription does affect your balance, ask your doctor if a similar product would work without causing dizziness.

Clean up clutter. Decorating is a matter of taste, but when it comes to fall prevention, less is best. Arrange your furniture and other belongings so you have plenty of room to move around, and don't put unnecessary objects on the floor.

Practice bathroom safety. Many serious falls happen in the bathroom, when you're all alone. Put bath mats or nonslip tape in

Help yourself to a full recovery

Recovering from a serious head injury can be a slow, difficult process. But recent research shows that your actions at home can make a difference to your recovery.

In a recent study, people with brain injuries were treated either in the hospital or at home. The home patients were taught strategies for improving their thinking and reasoning skills. They learned card and number games to exercise their brains. They also were encouraged to watch news programs and to read books and magazines.

The home-based patients recovered just as quickly and completely as people who went through a hospital program. Researchers suggest that a decreased stress level at home and the support of loved ones might be key factors in recovery.

your bathtub to prevent slipping, and use nonskid rugs on the floor. If you're unsteady getting in and out of the tub, install handrails to help.

Stay steady on the stairs. Staircases are another area where falls commonly occur. You should have a hand railing on both sides of any staircases in your home, and make sure you use them. If your stairs aren't carpeted, put nonslip treads on them, and make sure they're always clutter free and well lit.

Light your path. Your eyesight tends to worsen as you get older, making you more likely to stumble over items in dimly lit rooms. Lighten up those rooms, and install nightlights in bedrooms, hallways, bathrooms, and any other place you may visit in the night.

Keep it within reach. Arrange your cabinets with often-used items within easy reach. If you do have to get something that's stored above your head, use a sturdy stepstool, preferably one with handgrips. Never stand on a chair to reach overhead items.

Improve your balance. Regular exercise will keep your muscles in shape, make your bones stronger, and improve your balance. Tai chi is one type of exercise that is especially suited to seniors. This gentle form of martial art has been practiced for centuries by millions of Chinese. And a study at Emory University found that people 70 and older who took tai chi classes were half as likely to fall as before they took the classes. Contact your local recreation department, fitness club, or area hospital to see if they offer tai chi classes.

Protect your head. Are you an on-the-go type who enjoys more vigorous (and risky) activities than tai chi? If so, take Plassman's advice and protect your head. "I would suggest that individuals wear a protective helmet when they participate in activities that increase the risk of head injury such as bicycling, skate-boarding, roller-blading or riding a scooter," she says.

If you're careful, you may never have to deal with a head injury. But if you do, make sure your doctor knows about it, especially if it's one where you've lost consciousness. And if your memory is a problem now, be sure to tell him about any past head injuries, even if they happened years ago. In the study on World War II veterans, the injuries occurred 50 years earlier, so even accidents in the distant past could be a significant clue to your current health.

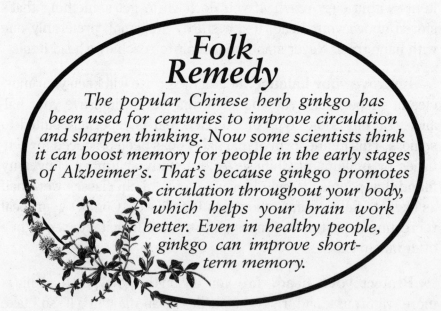

Folk
Remedy

The popular Chinese herb ginkgo has been used for centuries to improve circulation and sharpen thinking. Now some scientists think it can boost memory for people in the early stages of Alzheimer's. That's because ginkgo promotes circulation throughout your body, which helps your brain work better. Even in healthy people, ginkgo can improve short-term memory.

ANXIETY

Give stress the slip and save your health

You don't need a doctor to tell you stress isn't healthy, but you may need help learning to overcome it.

When you're dreading some event, you can feel your heart pounding, your hands sweating, and your head throbbing. If your tension is ongoing — say you're the caretaker of a sick relative — you might experience a sense of anxiety that never quite leaves. While all these sensations are certainly unpleasant, there's a darker, more dangerous side to stress.

- ↦ **Heart disease.** When you're under pressure, your heart takes a lot of abuse. The anxiety stress causes can lead to high blood pressure, atherosclerosis (hardening of your arteries), and abnormal heart rhythms.

- ↦ **Sleep disturbances.** You don't necessarily suffer from a sleep disorder or disease if you find yourself tossing and turning all

What is it?

It's normal to feel anxious when you're under stress. But if you're constantly nervous, worried, uneasy, or fearful, you may have an anxiety disorder. Some people have unexplainable feelings of dread every day. Others have specific fears called phobias that can keep them from living normally. You could also suffer from intense panic attacks that last anywhere from a couple of minutes to over an hour.

Symptoms:
- ↦ Dry mouth
- ↦ Sweating
- ↦ Irregular heartbeat
- ↦ Breathing difficulties
- ↦ Dizziness
- ↦ Stomach upset
- ↦ Muscle tension or trembling
- ↦ Insomnia
- ↦ Headaches

night. Too much daily pressure can disrupt your internal clock. Insomnia caused by stress can be fixed — but not with sleeping pills.

- **Weakened immune system.** Constant stress can affect your ability to fight sickness and leave you vulnerable to disease. You also may recover from surgery and wounds more slowly. Some researchers think stress might even damage your body's ability to repair cells — and lead to cancer.

- **Prostatitis.** Stressed-out men may suffer more from prostate disease than those who are relaxed. Anxiety triggers an increase in the hormone prolactin, which can cause prostate inflammation. And stress has been linked to high PSA (prostate-specific antigen), an indicator of increased prostate cancer risk.

- **Inflammatory bowel disease.** Studies show that while stress may not cause digestive diseases like Crohn's and ulcerative colitis, it can trigger attacks and make symptoms worse.

So now that you know you can make any medical treatment more effective by reducing stress, here's how to do it.

Bite into breakfast. Your mother always said it was the most important meal of the day, and she was right. Re-searchers in England found that breakfast eaters — who tend to have healthier lifestyles overall — have more energy and feel less stressed than those who skip breakfast. And cereal eaters feel better regardless of their other health habits. So, put some fuel in your tank before you start your hectic day.

Don't skimp on sleep. No matter how much you have to do, get at least eight hours of shut-eye. If anxiety keeps you from drifting off, don't stay in bed worrying. Get up, experts say, and do something relaxing — watch some mindless TV or look through a magazine. If your brain keeps racing, make a list of what's bothering you and then let it go until tomorrow.

Take a vacation. You dream of getting away, but all your responsibilities make it seem impossible. That's exactly why you should go. A relaxing vacation won't just renew you for a week or two. Interviews revealed vacationers felt better physically up to five weeks after a get-away.

If you're a full-time caretaker, you need time off on a regular basis to renew yourself. Find a relative or nursing service that can cover for a few weekends a month and occasionally for longer breaks.

Put on your gardening gloves. There's something soothing about digging in the dirt. Maybe it reminds you of days in the sandbox, or perhaps it just brings you closer to nature. However it works, gardening not only rewards you with a prettier yard but it also lets you get rid of some of those worries along with the weeds.

Karin Fleming, HTR, president of The American Horticultural Therapy Association, says, "Gardening is a great all-around exercise that can be enjoyed by people of all ages and abilities. It helps tone muscles, which promotes healthy bones, and it helps maintain flexibility, stamina, and strength. It is also a known fact that gardening helps reduce stress and lower blood pressure."

Laugh at life. You might not see anything funny about your hectic schedule, but try to find the humor in each situation — it will give you the opportunity to relieve a little tension. Experts say people who can laugh at difficulties deal better with stress and as a result suffer fewer health problems. Even renting a funny movie can help. So, start tuning in to the comedy around you. Instead of feeling as if life is out of control, you might start enjoying the show.

Forgive and forget. Holding a grudge is like holding yourself hostage. Anger and resentment can keep you from enjoying the good things in your life. When a group of men and women took a six-session course on forgiving others, they had fewer episodes of stress-related health problems. The health benefits of forgiveness were still obvious four months later at a follow-up session.

Massage your muscles. If you're keyed up, your muscles can feel tense and sore. A massage loosens those knots and helps you unwind and sleep better. Indulge.

Relax to music. Like taking a mini-vacation, listening to peaceful music can calm your nerves and ease muscle tension. Individual tastes will vary, but experts suggest giving classical music a try.

Write about it. Put your worries down on paper, and you might feel more in control of the situation. Some people believe keeping a journal helps them sort things out and identify possible solutions.

Get some sun. A sunny day can brighten your mood, but only if you get outside. Walk to the mailbox or a friend's house and the sunlight will boost your melatonin, a hormone that buffers the effects of stress and can help you sleep better.

Pray. If you believe in the power of prayer, you're not alone. In fact, for stress management and a general sense of well-being, seniors use prayer more than any other alternative treatment.

Having others pray for your health, even if you don't know about it, could speed your recovery. And if you're a caregiver, praying may help increase your ability to cope with stress.

Confide in a counselor. Sometimes you just need someone to help you sort things out. Counseling is a great way to get some expert advice when anxiety and stress feel overwhelming. Chances are good that your insurance will even cover it. Ask your doctor for a referral or confide in a trusted pastor, priest, or rabbi. Either way, you'll feel better after talking with someone who cares.

Soothe anxiety with these supplements

There might be trouble brewing in that pot of coffee — especially if you're feeling anxious already. Recent research suggests caffeine can trigger panic attacks and send your blood pressure through the roof. If you combine that with existing high blood pressure, the results can be serious. But don't despair. While you might have to say goodbye to caffeine, you can say hello to these natural stress busters.

Kava. A drink made from crushed kava roots plays an important role in Polynesian folk healing and cultural ceremonies. Because it produces a calming effect, kava should help in cases of mild to moderate anxiety, stress, or restlessness. However, follow dosage directions carefully since it might make you drowsy, and too much can be intoxicating. You can buy kava (also called kava kava) as a capsule, powder, extract, or ingredient in various herb drinks. The American Pharmaceutical Association says for anxiety take one or two 250-milligram capsules once or twice a day, but don't mix with alcohol.

Valerian. Like kava, valerian has been trusted to relieve tension for centuries. It's also a super sleep aid with no side effects. For valerian tea, add one teaspoon of the dried root to a cup of hot water. Or if you prefer, take three 475-milligram capsules three times a day.

ConsumerLab.com, an independent reviewer of dietary supplements and nutrition products, found that only half of the commercial valerian products they tested contained the amount of the herb they claimed to. When selecting a valerian product, look for the ConsumerLab.com Approved Quality Product Seal. At least you'll be getting what you paid for.

Ginseng. If you take ginseng, especially along with a multivitamin, you may recharge your adrenal gland, and so cope with stress better. Used in the Far East for thousands of years, this

Get a lift with aromatherapy

The research is out, and the verdict is in — aromatherapy can relieve tension and daily stress. To lift your spirits, experiment with these essential oils — bergamot, cedarwood, frankincense, geranium, hyssop, lavender, sandalwood, orange, and ylang ylang. Just remember, never place undiluted essential oils directly on your skin or in your mouth. Instead dilute them in water or "carrier oils" like almond, apricot, jojoba, and grapeseed.

- For the perfect massage, add 10 to 20 drops of essential oil to every one ounce of carrier oil.
- Get a steamy bath going and add five to 10 drops of essential oil and one ounce of carrier oil. Soak for at least 15 minutes.
- Dab a handkerchief with three to four drops of your favorite oil. Whenever and wherever stress strikes, sniff it at arm's length for instant relief.
- For a stress headache, soak a hand towel in a mixture of a half-cup of water and five to 10 drops of oil. Hold the compress to your forehead until the towel is cold.
- A 10-minute footbath with hot water and a few drops of essential oil, especially lavender, will make you feel pampered and peaceful.

healing root also boosts energy and concentration. Ginseng is available in several forms, including capsules, teas, soft drinks, dried root, and even chewing gum.

Chamomile. Brew a soothing cup of chamomile tea by steeping two or three teaspoons of dried blossoms in a cup of water. Then sit back and sip your anxieties away.

Vitamin C. Your brain needs vitamin C to produce serotonin, a chemical that helps you sleep and makes you feel good. Without enough, you may feel tired and sluggish. When you're under a lot of stress, this vitamin will also block the release of stress hormones that weaken your immune system. It will help if you remember C is for "Calm."

Energize yourself with this wonderful vitamin by eating citrus fruits, strawberries, red and green peppers, broccoli, Brussels sprouts, and cantaloupe. For more protection, take vitamin C supplements.

B vitamins. Getting enough B vitamins in your diet is essential during times of anxiety because your body uses them quickly when it's stressed. If you don't get the right amount, you can actually develop depression and tension. Vitamins B12, B5 (pantothenic acid), and folate are especially important. Eat peas, beans, meat, poultry, fish, whole-grain breads and cereals, bananas, and potatoes for the important Bs. Or look for them in a multivitamin.

Magnesium. A Yugoslavian study found that people exposed to chronic stress had lower magnesium levels. To make sure you get plenty of this important mineral, especially during stressful times, eat beans, brown rice, grains, popcorn, nuts, spinach, peas, corn, potatoes, oatmeal, shrimp, clams, oysters, and skim milk. Supplements are also available if you can't fit enough magnesium into your diet. But be careful — too much magnesium can be dangerous.

SAM-e. Pronounced "sammy," this friendly little biochemical (full name S-adenosylmethionine) has been used in Europe for decades and is finally gaining popularity in the United States. Not only does it show promise as an arthritis treatment, but it might also treat depression and anxiety just as well as prescription antidepressants — without the unpleasant side effects. Ask your doctor about this super supplement.

When exercise won't lower stress

You work on the loading dock of a major trucking firm. Between the long hours and impossible deadlines, you're constantly under stress. You know the tension's not good for your heart, but you've heard exercise lowers stress. With all that lifting and hauling, surely things must balance out. Unfortunately, at least one expert says not to count on it.

"If you think being physically active at work is helping your heart, think again if you also have workplace stress," advises Dr. James H. Dwyer of the University of Southern California's Keck School of Medicine.

Dwyer and his fellow researchers studied the effects of physical activity — at the job site and during free time away from work — on a group of workers for a utility company. The study took place at a time when workers faced stressful adjustments due to deregulation.

At the beginning of the study, researchers used ultrasound to measure the thickness of the workers' carotid arteries — a strong indicator of heart disease. None of them had atherosclerosis, a build-up of cholesterol-rich plaque in their blood vessels. When they measured again three years later, they were surprised by the results.

Employees that got the most physical activity on the job had almost twice as much plaque build-up in their carotid arteries as those who got very little exercise at work. On the other hand, those who exercised at least four times per week during their leisure time had the smallest increase and, therefore, the healthiest arteries of all.

On further investigation, the researchers discovered that workers who did the most physical labor were also more likely to report poor sleep and other symptoms of stress.

Having little control over work conditions can contribute to feelings of anxiety. "It was not so much the danger of the job," says Dwyer, "as it was the demands of the job, the uncertainties, the difficulties working with other people. These are the kinds of stresses that develop in any workplace."

So, whether or not your job requires physical activity, protect your heart by exercising regularly in your free time — hiking, biking, swimming, or gardening. In addition, here are some things you can do at work to lower stress.

Practice deep breathing. Most people take 12 to 15 shallow breaths per minute. Slowing it down to about eight per minute can calm you, slow your heart rate, and give you more energy.

Breathe through your nose and fill your lungs completely. Let your diaphragm fall so low it pushes out your abdomen — as if you were breathing into your stomach. Exhale slowly, releasing all the air, while staying relaxed.

Take rewarding breaks from work. Listen to pleasant music or talk about something enjoyable when you take a time-out. Avoid people who spend this time complaining and you're less likely to feel drained and tense when you return to your responsibilities.

Move in a different way. Get away from your workstation now and then and do a physical activity unrelated to your work. Take a walk, do some stretching, or practice a bit of yoga or tai chi.

These practices should make your work life more enjoyable. What's more, you'll increase the chances that when you're ready for the pleasures of retirement your heart will be going strong.

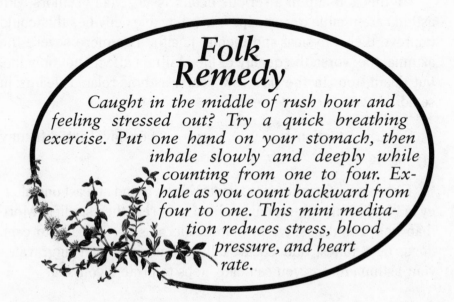

Folk
Remedy

Caught in the middle of rush hour and feeling stressed out? Try a quick breathing exercise. Put one hand on your stomach, then inhale slowly and deeply while counting from one to four. Exhale as you count backward from four to one. This mini meditation reduces stress, blood pressure, and heart rate.

ASTHMA

Take breathing troubles seriously

Shortness of breath doesn't mean you're getting long in the tooth. It could mean you have asthma. Contrary to popular belief, many people suffer their first asthma attack after age 70. Here's another surprise — often, this asthma is due to allergies.

If you're a senior, you may not be diagnosed with asthma because you have heart or lung disease, health problems that can mask the condition. And, according to a recent Canadian study, even if you are diagnosed, you might not get the best medication for your condition — inhaled steroids.

All this adds up to a serious health issue. Many seniors with asthma are unable to participate in enjoyable activities that could improve their physical and mental health. The more severe the asthma, the worse the quality of life. Asthma affects not only life, but death, too. In the past few years, asthma-related deaths in seniors have gone up 24 percent.

So, pay attention if you or someone you love has difficulty breathing.

Get tested for allergies. Researchers found at least one allergy in 75 percent of the senior asthma sufferers they studied. More than half tested positive to indoor allergies — typically to cats, dogs, dust mites, and cockroaches. Knowing what aggravates your asthma means you can take steps to protect yourself.

Put your house to rights. If you do have allergies, start making your home more asthma-friendly. This might mean giving up furry pets like cats and dogs, storing away stuffed animals, removing plants, or encasing your mattress in plastic. Keep things clean — dust and vacuum regularly. Think about replacing your carpet with wood or vinyl floors. If you live in an older home or collect antiques, you're probably living with more dust. High humidity and bedrooms that stay above 70 degrees both encourage the growth of mold.

Ask about medication. Inhaled steroids slash hospitalization in half and deaths by 90 percent. Unfortunately, in a Canadian study, 40 percent of seniors with asthma did not get a prescription for them. Ask your doctor about inhaled steroids and make sure you understand how to use them. Researchers found half of seniors used their inhaler regularly, whether they needed to or not, instead of only during an asthma attack. This means many people need better long-term medication to treat their asthma.

Advice from your doctor about timing is also important. According to the American Medical Association, your risk of an asthma attack is highest at night. Ask your doctor about sustained-release bronchodilators. These pills can take up to an hour to start working, but they'll open up your lungs for 12 to 24 hours. Take them in the evening so they'll be most effective when your asthma symptoms hit.

Find a specialist. Many times, general practitioners won't treat asthma as aggressively as a specialist will. If your asthma isn't getting

---

What is it?

Asthmatics have airways that overreact to different triggers. During an attack, the muscles of the walls of your bronchi — the air passageways between your lungs and trachea — spasm and swell. The airways close up and you have trouble breathing, especially breathing out. Allergies are the biggest trigger for asthma, but some people have asthma attacks when exercising or when under stress. Some cases of asthma don't seem to have any obvious trigger.

Symptoms:
- Wheezing
- Difficulty breathing
- Coughing
- Tightness in chest
- Anxiety

the proper attention, seek out an allergist who understands your condition and is willing to try the latest, most effective treatments.

Fend off asthma with your knife and fork

A restaurant worker, sensitive to seafood, simply breathed in the vapor of cooking shrimp and scallops and set off his asthma. This is one case of food working against you. With asthma, it's important to learn which foods are your friends and which mean trouble.

Stay away from sulfites. Many alcoholic drinks, especially wine, contain sulfites and salicylates. These chemical preservatives keep food and beverages from spoiling, but they can quickly trigger an asthma attack in sensitive people. If you have a reaction like this to wine, other sulfite-containing foods, like shrimp and salad bar items, will probably affect your breathing, as well.

Remember to choose your pain and cold medications with care. Aspirin and other nonsteroidal anti-inflammatory drugs contain allergy-triggering salicylates. Not only can they bring on an asthma attack, they have been named the culprit in at least a few cases of another serious lung condition — pneumonia. Talk to your doctor about what over-the-counter medications you can safely take.

Forgo fast food. Maybe they should call it "fat food." The typical fast-food meal has too much saturated fat, too many calories, and too little nutrition. Eating too much of it is also linked to asthma and wheezing. If you make the switch to healthier foods, not only can you reduce your risk of breathing problems, but you could also lose that spare tire which is especially hard on your lungs. Studies show weight loss can improve lung function and allow you to use less asthma medication.

So, never mind how convenient that drive-thru is, or how much you like the taste. You'll like taking a deep breath even better.

Opt for omega-3. Corn, cotton, and safflower oils; dressings; mayonnaise; margarine; and processed foods are all full of omega-6 fatty acids. These can make inflammatory diseases and asthma worse. However, foods with omega-3 fatty acids have the opposite effect. Good sources are leafy green vegetables; cold-water fish like salmon, mackerel, and tuna; and flaxseed oil, which you can buy at most health food stores. Refrigerate flaxseed oil since it spoils quickly and don't cook with it. But you can use it on salads and in baked goods. For cooking oil, try canola, which has a good balance of omega-3 and omega-6 oils.

Maneuver around asthma attacks

When someone is choking on food, you probably know what to do. But if someone has an asthma attack, you might stand by helplessly. Fortunately, what works for choking also works for asthma — the Heimlich Maneuver.

According to the Heimlich Institute, the famous anti-choking action works by forcing trapped air and mucus out of the lungs. The Heimlich Maneuver, if performed regularly, might even prevent future asthma attacks.

Here's how to perform the Heimlich Maneuver on someone suffering from a life-threatening asthma attack.

- Stand behind the choker and wrap your arms around his waist.
- Make a fist, and place the thumb side of that fist against the upper abdomen, above the belly button but below the ribcage.
- Grab your fist with your other hand and press into the upper abdomen with a quick, but gentle upward thrust. Do not squeeze the ribcage.
- Repeat if necessary.

If you're alone and having an asthma attack, you can perform the Heimlich Maneuver on yourself. Just skip the first step and follow the rest of the directions. Or you can lean over a table, chair, or railing and briefly force your upper abdomen against its edge.

Develop an appetite for apples. Apples get an "A" when it comes to asthma relief. Eating five or more every week may improve how well your lungs function. Experts think a mix of antioxidants — especially quercetin — could protect your lungs from tissue damage. Try having an apple each day for a delicious, low-calorie snack.

Eat more E. Vitamin E is a powerful antioxidant that can help protect your body — including your lungs — from free radical damage. For a natural supply of vitamin E, eat sweet potatoes, fortified cereals, and sunflower seeds. Or take a supplement of not more than 400 international units (IU). More can cause diarrhea, dizziness, and other side effects.

Have a jolt of java. There's no better way to start your morning than taking in the rich aroma of brewing coffee. But your lungs can benefit from a cup even more than your nose — especially if you suffer from asthma. The chemical makeup of caffeine is similar to the commonly prescribed asthma drug theophylline. That means caffeine can help expand your air passages and keep your respiratory muscles strong. Just a couple cups of coffee can help you breathe better for up to four hours.

Attack asthma with a killer tomato

The antioxidant lycopene, found in tomatoes, has received top billing lately as a cancer-fighter. Now it looks like lycopene can also help defeat a kind of asthma that hits when you're trying to exercise.

Regular exercise can keep you in shape and increase your heart and lungpower — benefits most asthma sufferers could really use. But exercise-induced asthma, or EIA, is the curse of many asthmatics who work out for stronger lungs and actually end up triggering an asthma attack. What's a wheezer to do?

In a recent study, people with EIA were given 30 milligrams (mg) of lycopene every day for a week. More than half showed fewer exercise-induced asthma symptoms. The enriched lycopene product they received, LYC-O-MATO™, also contained other antioxidants such as vitamin E. Although researchers believe lycopene could take most of the credit for reducing EIA, the combination of antioxidants may have played a role.

You can get 30 mg of lycopene from just over a cup of tomato juice, or from about half a cup of spaghetti sauce. Increase your daily dose of lycopene by pouring a little extra ketchup on your burger and adding tomatoes to sandwiches and salads. Remember, eating a variety of fruits and vegetables will give you plenty of other antioxidants, as well.

Another way to beat EIA is to drink lots of liquids. A study presented to the American College of Sports Medicine showed that dehydrated asthmatics have much more trouble with EIA than those who take in plenty of fluids. For powerful asthma prevention, combine these two remedies by reaching for juicy fruits that contain lots of water and lycopene. Watermelon, guava, and pink grapefruit are good choices.

Make these minor adjustments to your eating habits, and you might find yourself breathing instead of wheezing during exercise.

Beware what you breathe

Take a deep breath. Feels good, doesn't it? When you have asthma, you appreciate every good breath you can get. But sometimes the air itself is polluted with unseen chemicals that cause serious breathing problems. Don't be caught off guard by these hidden asthma triggers.

Forget the fireworks. That funny smell in the air after a fireworks explosion comes from sulfur dioxide and other chemicals. These can irritate your lungs, especially if you have asthma.

A hospital in Philadelphia reported two cases of asthmatic children suffering severe attacks while playing with fireworks. A 13-year-old boy survived, but a 9-year-old girl with moderate asthma didn't. She had only been playing with sparklers — something most people consider harmless.

Doctors warn asthmatics, and especially children, to be careful during fireworks demonstrations. Luckily, you can see them from a distance, so there's no need to miss the fun. If you have asthma, stay far away from the cloud of chemicals given off during the explosion. And asthma sufferers should probably avoid hand-held fireworks altogether.

Don't dive into trouble. Jumping into a cool swimming pool on a hot day is usually refreshing. But if the water is treated with chlorine, and you have asthma, watch out. You could be inhaling tiny chlorine particles that can trigger breathing problems. In a recent survey of competitive swimmers, half had asthma symptoms, most likely due to their constant exposure to chlorine.

At the first sign of wheezing or shortness of breath, get out of the water. And if you have asthma symptoms every time you swim, you might need to switch to another form of exercise.

Watch out for workplace contaminants. Researchers report one in 10 asthmatics suffer attacks because of a trigger in their work environment. The air might seem perfectly fine, but it could contain dust, fumes, gasses, and chemicals. If you're a carpenter, concrete worker, drug manufacturer, printer, food process worker, spray painter, or electrician, you're at an increased risk.

See your doctor if you think your job is making you sick. Typical symptoms are wheezing, coughing, or shortness of breath that may happen just at work, or a few hours after you leave. Test it out by seeing how you feel on vacation or on weekends. If your breathing problems clear up, the source may be at work. According to the American Lung Association, the only way to truly beat occupational asthma is to switch jobs.

Guard against gas fumes. Do you wheeze while you're fixing dinner? If your stove uses gas, there may be a logical explanation. Gas gives off nitrogen dioxide, a pollutant. Researchers have found that people who cook with gas stoves are at least twice as likely to develop breathing problems like asthma. If your kitchen causes you to cough, it may be time to trade in for an electric stove.

Alternative therapies ease asthma symptoms

Telling someone who's having an asthma attack to relax is kind of like telling someone who just wrecked his new car to smile. The breathlessness of an asthma attack just naturally causes panic and tension. Still, relaxing is exactly what you need to do since tense muscles are only going to make your attack worse. Try these alternative therapies to help you gain some breathing space.

Breathe better. If you have asthma, you'll breathe easier by learning to breathe differently. According to a recent survey, many asthmatics have tried breathing techniques, and most found the exercises helpful. Psychologist and breathing expert Dr. Gay Hendricks says everyone can improve the way he breathes. His book, *Conscious Breathing: Breathwork for Health, Stress Release, and Personal Mastery,* contains exercises designed specifically for people with asthma. Here are some general tips.

- **Breathe through your nose.** Dust and other irritants can trigger an asthma attack. While it can't keep out all trouble, your nose is designed to filter out some of these pollutants. Let it be your first line of defense.

- **Take it slow.** Most people breathe too rapidly, making their lungs and their hearts work too hard. Concentrate on slowing your breathing down to about 8 to 12 breaths per minute.

- **Go deep.** To make sure air reaches the lowest part of your lungs, take deep breaths, pushing your diaphragm down into your abdomen.

- **Empty your lungs fully.** Most people with asthma probably don't empty their lungs completely when they breathe out, perhaps because they fear they'll never get another good breath. But if you pull your abdomen in tightly when you exhale, you'll push all the old air out and have plenty of room for fresh air on your next breath.

- **Stay in your comfort zone.** Breathing exercises are designed to relax, not make you more stressed. Don't push yourself to breathe too deeply or slowly at first. With a little practice, good breathing will be a breeze.

Imagine a solution. Some asthmatics find that visualizing a comforting image during an asthma attack helps them breathe easier.

- Get in a comfortable position, either sitting or reclining.

- Close your eyes and gradually relax your muscles, beginning with your toes and working your way up.

- Imagine a scene that you find relaxing. Although this process is often called visualization, you can use all your senses. If you find a beach scene relaxing, don't just imagine what it looks like — imagine how the salt air smells, hear the sound of waves lapping at the shore, and feel the moist air and warm sun on your face.

Take a breather with yoga. In 1984, an accident at a Union Carbide plant in India exposed millions to toxic gas, leaving some with chronic asthma symptoms. Recently, researchers reported that yoga helped many find relief.

Another study in Colorado found that asthmatics practicing yoga techniques were more relaxed, had a better attitude, and tended to use their inhalers less.

Yoga typically involves breathing exercises (pranayama), physical postures (yogasanas), and meditation. While yoga won't eliminate asthma, all three aspects may help you control your symptoms. To find a yoga instructor in your area, contact your local recreation department, YMCA, or fitness center.

Practice prayer. According to research, older people use prayer to control stress more than any other alternative therapy. Science even supports the power of prayer to heal. If praying helps relax you during an asthma attack, by all means, pray. There are no known side effects.

Keep in mind these relaxing therapies should be used in addition to — not instead of — your asthma medication.

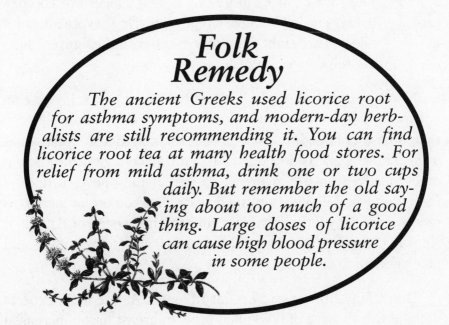

Folk Remedy

The ancient Greeks used licorice root for asthma symptoms, and modern-day herbalists are still recommending it. You can find licorice root tea at many health food stores. For relief from mild asthma, drink one or two cups daily. But remember the old saying about too much of a good thing. Large doses of licorice can cause high blood pressure in some people.

BREAST CANCER

Don't overestimate your risk

The statistics are enough to send cold chills down your spine. One in nine American women will develop breast cancer. So you wonder, does that mean for every group of nine women, one will be stricken with breast cancer?

Only if the nine women are randomly selected and have their entire lives ahead of them, which means newborn babies. Your risk as an older woman is actually much lower. For example, during your 50s, your chances of getting breast cancer are approximately 1 in 30 because you have already survived several decades of risk. While you are right to be concerned with the figures, don't overestimate the danger.

Know your family risk. It wasn't too long ago that breast cancer was a taboo subject, not fit for polite conversation. Luckily, things have changed. If your extended family doesn't talk about such things, start asking questions. You have a right to know if other relatives have had breast cancer. If they have, it doesn't mean you will definitely get the disease, but you are at increased risk — especially if the relative is your mother, sister, or daughter. Knowing your family risk can help you stay alert to symptoms and take prevention seriously.

Don't fear fibrocystic breast disease. At one time, experts thought this disease of fluid-filled cysts in breast tissue increased your chances of cancer. Now they believe there is no connection. But if your doctor says you have a proliferative breast disease, your risk is somewhat higher.

Ignore the rumor of the week. It's bad enough how fast rumors can spread by word of mouth, but now rumors can instantly reach millions by way of the Internet. Have you heard that antiperspirants cause breast cancer? Not true. Neither is the one about mammograms causing cancer. Base your beliefs on facts supported by science, and leave the rumors to the tabloids.

Practice prevention. Instead of worrying — which won't protect you — take the following measures that could.

- ✧ **Monthly self-exam.** Ask your doctor to show you how to do a self-exam. Check your breasts the week after your period or, if you're past menopause, the first of every month. Do the exam faithfully, and call your doctor if you find any unusual changes in skin texture, color, or shape. Also, watch for any swelling, pain, or discharge from a nipple. And, of course, report any suspicious lump or thickening of breast tissue.

- ✧ **Yearly mammogram at 40.** Mammograms can be a little uncomfortable, but here's a statistic that makes the discomfort more than worth it. Your chances of surviving breast cancer jump to 95 percent with early

---

What is it?

When cells in your body change and multiply without control, they can spread and eventually overrun healthy cells. This is called cancer. Breast cancer often starts with a small lump in your breast. Since you usually can't see tumors, monthly breast self-exams are vital. Most lumps women find in their breasts are NOT cancerous, but breast cancer that is not caught and treated early is usually fatal. By the time a tumor is three-quarters of an inch wide, it may have spread cancer to other parts of your body.

Symptoms:
- ✧ Lump in or around breast
- ✧ Thickened breast tissue
- ✧ Breast pain
- ✧ Wrinkled or puckered skin
- ✧ Nipple discharge
- ✧ Change in nipple size or appearance

detection. These radiographic pictures can find tiny changes in your breasts that you might not notice for several more years.

- **Healthy diet.** Experts think you can reduce your risk up to 50 percent by eating plenty of fruits, whole grains, and vegetables and by going easy on fats and sweets. Maintaining a healthy body weight, especially after menopause, will also increase the odds in your favor.

- **Limit alcohol.** One drink a day is the maximum you should allow yourself if you're serious about avoiding breast cancer. If the disease runs in your family, consider not drinking at all.

- **Exercise.** After checking with your doctor, add some sort of workout to your daily routine — even walking will do — and aim for 45 minutes to an hour. Choose something you enjoy so you'll stick with it. At least once a week, work up a sweat and get your heart going for about an hour.

- **Regular checkups.** If you're between 20 and 39, have your doctor examine your breasts every three years or so. She may opt to check more often depending on your history. After 40, you should have annual breast exams. If a lump is detected, don't panic. Most lumps are not cancerous. And remember, if cancer rears its ugly head, early detection is your best defense.

Winning the breast cancer battle

You looked into the eyes of the monster called breast cancer, and after your initial terror, you decided to fight. Because you are determined to survive, you will use every weapon you can find.

If your cancer was detected early, time is on your side. But no matter when you received the shocking diagnosis, how well and how long you live depends on more than the drugs you take. This year alone about 182,000 women will be told they have breast cancer, and many will die. But researchers have found that breast cancer survivors tend to have certain attitudes and behaviors in common. You can fight the good fight with these proven weapons.

Control stress. A recent survey of breast cancer survivors found that more of them blamed stress for causing their cancer than anything else. But according to researchers, other factors — such as genetics, environment, diet, and hormones — are much more likely to affect your breast cancer risk.

Nevertheless, the way you deal with stress may have an effect on your surviving breast cancer. One study found that women with breast cancer who learned how to manage stress had lower levels of the stress hormone cortisol, which is known to suppress your immune system. They also had higher levels of an antibody to mucin, a chemical associated with breast cancer. In addition, they were more likely to finish their full course of chemotherapy because they experienced fewer problems, such as nausea and vomiting. All of these things could have a significant effect on survival.

Express your emotions. Breast cancer can flood you with an ocean of emotions, and how you deal with those feelings could have a big impact on your survival. In one study, women with breast cancer who coped by expressing their emotions had more energy, less distress, and fewer medical appointments for cancer-related problems.

In another study, women with breast cancer who expressed their emotions and had adequate emotional support had a survival rate two to four times higher than other women.

So don't put on a brave front for your family and friends. Tell them how you're feeling and accept their support and sympathy.

You may live longer, and they'll feel that they were important to your recovery.

Get more exercise. Research shows that regular exercise may help you avoid breast cancer. But even if you weren't active before having the disease, it's not too late to start. In the early stages of breast cancer treatment, exercise may help you combat the fatigue often caused by treatment. And a recent study found that women with breast cancer who exercised regularly reported having a higher quality of life than those who didn't exercise.

Watch what you eat. Experts disagree on whether eating a low-fat diet helps prevent breast cancer, but eating less saturated fat and more fruits, vegetables, and whole grains will improve your health overall. And since obesity is a risk factor for breast cancer, maintaining a healthy weight may help prevent recurrences. One study revealed that women who consumed a diet high in protein, which included poultry, fish, and dairy products — but not red meat, were more likely to survive breast cancer.

Researchers have focused much attention on the diet of the people living around the Mediterranean Sea. These people live longer and suffer fewer diseases than in other parts of the world. But instead of one or two special foods, the benefits probably come from the variety of healthy, plant-based foods they eat.

Dr. Mariette Gerber, head of the Metabolic Epidemiology Group at the French Institute of Health and Medical Research in Montpellier, France, says, "There is a distressing tendency for people to oversimplify what we have come to know about diets of the Mediterranean region. People say, 'Oh, it's the red wine,' or 'It's the olive oil,' or 'It's the fish,' when the truth is significantly more complex." Dr. Gerber says it is all of these things working together and more.

So strive for diversity when you fill your plate with healthy foods. Go easy on the red meats and keep adding new plant foods to your diet.

Keep yourself informed. An interesting new study points to the possibility that breast cancer victims with high levels of insulin in their blood seem to be more likely to die of the disease than other women. Insulin, which promotes normal cell growth, also encourages the growth of cancer cells in the breast. Experts say it's still too early to start monitoring insulin levels in women who have breast cancer. More studies are necessary.

Don't delay treatment. Why would a woman put off treatment that could save her life? Fear might play a role in the decision to wait. But researchers came up with some other reasons. For example, a recent death in the family made women seven times more likely to delay treatment for breast cancer. In addition, women under constant stress, and those involved with people critical of them, were more apt to delay treatment.

Remember, you're in a battle, and retreat is not an option. In order to survive breast cancer, you must get medical attention immediately. If you feel you're not important enough, see a counselor to help you sort out your feelings and to learn to deal with negative people. But start medical treatment at once. You can win this battle, but only if you fight.

Find strength in sharing. The practices that improve your odds against cancer can be applied to any disease. Encourage others to take these same healthy steps in facing their illnesses, and you'll strengthen your own resolve.

Eat well and avoid breast cancer

If you're a woman who lives in North America or Western Europe, you're six to 10 times more likely to develop breast cancer than women in Japan and other less-developed areas of the world. Scientists aren't sure what accounts for this higher rate of the disease in certain countries, but some believe it's linked to diet. Asian women who move to the United States increase their risk of breast cancer, perhaps because they adopt an American style of eating.

Dr. David Heber, Chair and co-founder of the Center for Human Nutrition at UCLA, recommends a diet of variety and moderation for cancer prevention.

"The weight of evidence is convincing," he says, "that a diet rich in a variety of vegetables, fruits, whole grains, and beans helps reduce cancer risk among individuals who have never had cancer. There are no guarantees, of course. But these foods do contain potent vitamins, minerals, and phytochemicals that seem to come to the body's aid to fight against and even halt the cancer process."

Fill up on fruits and veggies. Fruits and vegetables may be low on the food chain, but they top the list of healthy foods to eat. The National Cancer Institute recommends that you eat at least five servings of fruits and vegetables every day. They base their recommendation on research pointing to the cancer preventive powers of fruits and vegetables.

In one large study, women who ate two or more servings of fruits and vegetables daily were 17 percent less likely to develop breast cancer than those who ate less than one serving of fruits and vegetables a day. And in another study, women who ate the recommended five servings a day reduced their risk of breast cancer by a whopping 54 percent compared with women who ate less than three daily servings.

And yet, not all fruits and vegetables have equal benefits. According to research, vegetables may be more protective than fruits, and raw vegetables may provide more benefits than cooked vegetables. When you're choosing the best vegetables for breast cancer protection, think color. Deep orange or yellow vegetables, such as carrots and squash, and dark green vegetables, such as spinach and broccoli, may be especially beneficial.

Go for the green. Vegetables aren't the only green source of breast cancer protection. Research shows drinking green tea regularly may reduce your risk of breast cancer, as well as other types of cancer.

Green tea contains powerful antioxidants that scientists credit for its ability to chase away cancer. One study in Japan found that green tea reduced the risk of all types of cancers, particularly among women who drank 10 or more cups a day. Another study found that women with breast cancer who drank more than five cups of green tea a day were less likely to have a recurrence of the disease. So if you're hoping to prevent breast cancer, help yourself to a soothing cup of green tea often.

Get the facts on fat. Researchers have focused much attention on the role of dietary fat in breast cancer. That's because breast cancer rates and fat intake are both higher in the United States than in other countries. Women in the United States typically get about 30 to 40 percent of their calories from fat. In areas where the breast cancer rate is lower, such as Asia, women may only get about 15 to 20 percent of their calories from fat.

Early studies supported the idea that eating too much fat could increase your risk of breast cancer, but more recent studies have not been able to confirm that. Obesity does increase your risk of breast cancer, however, and eating too much fat can contribute to weight gain.

The kind of fat you eat could make a difference, too. In Mediterranean countries, the total fat intake is as high as in the United States, yet breast cancer rates are lower. That could be because the main source of fat for people there is olive oil, which is a monounsaturated fat. Some studies have found that olive oil is slightly protective against breast cancer.

While there are no clear answers yet on how fat affects breast cancer, eating low fat is still a healthy choice. Limit your intake of saturated fats, which come mostly from animal products such as butter, red meat, and whole milk. Try to use oils low in saturated fats, such as olive oil and canola oil, instead.

Load up on fiber. Filling your plate with fiber instead of fat could also protect you from breast cancer. Lower estrogen levels are associated with a reduced risk of breast cancer, and research shows that fiber reduces circulating estrogen levels in pre-menopausal women, although it may not reduce the already low levels of estrogen in postmenopausal women.

You can increase your fiber intake by eating more fruits and vegetables — also believed to be protective against breast cancer. Whole grains offer another good source of fiber. Most studies have found that fiber from whole grains is slightly protective against breast cancer, but some studies have found no effect. Either way, eating more grains will provide healthy variety to your diet, and that's just what the doctor ordered.

Simple bone test can predict your risk

Strong bones are less likely to break — and broken bones are a real concern for older women. Unfortunately, a new study has found that having strong bones might also mean you're more likely to develop breast cancer — another concern for older women.

Researchers tested bone density in almost 9,000 women age 65 and older and then tracked them for about six years to see who developed breast cancer. Those with the highest bone density were almost three times more likely to develop breast cancer than women with the lowest bone density.

Estrogen probably accounts for the connection between the two conditions. High levels of estrogen are associated with both higher bone density and a higher risk of breast cancer. Researchers stress that dense bones don't cause breast cancer, but bone density testing might provide a new way for doctors to identify women who are at high risk for the disease.

If your bone mineral density test comes back with a high reading, talk with your doctor about breast cancer prevention and screening, but don't stop doing things that make your bones strong, such as exercising and eating foods high in calcium. Yogurt, sardines, milk, and turnip greens are excellent sources.

CATARACTS

Nutritional ABCs that will save your sight

Cataracts strike nearly everyone by age 75. But just by eating the right things — and avoiding the harmful ones — you can protect yourself from cataracts and other vision problems.

Ante up with vitamin A. The first of three protective antioxidant vitamins gets top billing when it comes to helping your eyes. Vitamin A guards against free radical damage that can lead to night blindness, cataracts, and macular degeneration. High doses of vitamin A have even been used to successfully treat a rare genetic eye disorder called Sorsby's fundus dystrophy, which can cause blindness.

Meats and dairy products contain vitamin A, but your body converts plant substances called carotenoids — such as beta carotene, lutein, and zeaxanthin — into vitamin A as well. Choose bright yellow or orange fruits and vegetables like apricots, carrots, and sweet potatoes for beta carotene. Green, leafy vegetables like spinach and collard greens give you plenty of lutein and zeaxanthin.

Be smart about B vitamins. It's not just the antioxidant vitamins that protect your eyes. The Blue Mountain Eye Study discovered that people deficient in the B vitamins niacin, thiamin, and riboflavin were more likely to get nuclear cataracts, the kind that affects the central part of your lens. Eating a bowl of fortified breakfast cereal will give you all three of these key nutrients.

Other sources include tuna, whole-wheat bread, baked potatoes, and mushrooms.

See better with C. Vitamin C, another antioxidant, also plays a role in protecting your eyes from free radicals. Oranges, lemons, tangerines, strawberries, cantaloupe, broccoli, brussels sprouts, and sweet red peppers are all rich sources of vitamin C.

Eat enough E. A full dose of vitamin E every day can cut your risk of getting cataracts in half. Just like vitamin A, vitamin E counteracts the harmful free radicals produced by exposure to light and oxygen. You can find E in wheat germ, sunflower seeds, nuts, whole grains, and brown rice.

Pay attention to protein. Chances are, you get enough protein from the meat, fish, and dairy products in your diet. But a protein deficiency could put you at greater risk for nuclear cataracts. If you're a vegetarian, this is a real concern. Make sure you mix your vegetable proteins — which are "incomplete" by themselves — to maximize your protection. For example, eat beans with rice and enjoy peanut butter with whole-grain bread.

> ### *What is it?*
>
> When the lens in your eye becomes permanently cloudy instead of clear, you have a cataract. It develops gradually over the years, slowly blurring your vision and turning colors dull. You may experience double vision and become sensitive to light. In time, your lens looks yellowish or milky-white. If left untreated, you could become blind.
>
> Symptoms:
> - Distorted vision
> - Cloudy appearance of lens
> - Poor night vision
> - Eye pain (in advanced cases)

Spare the salt. A high-salt diet could mean high risk for your eyes. In fact, in one study, those whose diet included about 3,000 milligrams (mg) of salt a day were twice as likely to develop cataracts as those getting only about 1,000 mg a day.

Try using herbs instead of salt to flavor your food. Garlic and onions improve almost any meal, and turmeric might even improve

8 little-known causes of cataracts

Over 50 percent of people ages 65 to 75 have cataracts. After age 75, that number shoots to 70 percent. Everyone knows a lifetime of exposure to sunlight, smoking, and drinking increases your odds of becoming a part of this statistic. But you might not be aware of these other major risk factors for cataracts.

- diabetes
- family history of cataracts
- atopic dermatitis, a persistent skin rash marked by patches of irritated, red skin
- poor diet, especially one short on antioxidants
- damage to the eye caused by a blunt or sharp object
- certain medications, like corticosteroid therapy
- exposure to radiation
- electrical shock

your eyesight. This spice, often used in Indian curry dishes, contains curcumin, an antioxidant that helped fight off cataracts in animal studies.

Also, avoid fast foods and read the labels before buying processed items, which are often high in sodium.

Junk the junk. Fat, alcohol, and cigarettes each increases your risk for cataracts. Together they are a devastating combination. Choose lean meats and low-fat dairy products and avoid cooking with saturated fats like lard, butter, and coconut oil. Limit yourself to no more than one or two drinks a day, and put out those cigarettes.

Protecting your vision doesn't have to be complicated. As you plan your meals from day to day, just remember, how you eat affects how you see.

Top-selling herb may cause cataracts

St. John's wort, sometimes called "herbal Prozac," may be making you more susceptible to cataracts.

In some people, St. John's wort acts as a photosensitizer, making you more sensitive to the effects of sunlight. And that can increase your chances of developing cataracts.

Many prescription drugs can also increase your sensitivity to sunlight, including antihistamines, antibiotics, and nonsteroidal anti-inflammatory drugs, such as ibuprofen. Fortunately, not everyone who takes these medicines will have a reaction — it depends on the individual.

Short-term effects of photosensitization include mild allergic reactions, hives, itching, rashes, eye burn, and increased susceptibility to sunburn. Long-term exposure to photosensitizers can lead to more severe allergic reactions, premature skin aging, skin cancer, and a weakened immune system, in addition to an increased risk of cataracts.

Because of the potentially serious side effects, find out if any drugs or supplements you're taking may be photosensitizers before you head outdoors. And, although experts aren't certain if sunscreen and sunglasses can prevent these side effects, it's always a good idea to protect yourself from the sun's damaging rays.

COLD AND FLU

Get your body into flu-fighting shape

Influenza is no minor illness. Up to 300,000 people a year land in the hospital because of it. Even more frightening, as many as 40,000 of them die.

If you're a senior, or have a serious heart or lung disease, you're at the greatest risk for coming down with a dangerous case of the flu. That's because your immune system might not be strong enough on its own to fend off the infection. But like a heavyweight boxer in training, you can get your body into prime flu-fighting shape. Start by pumping up your immune system with these training tips, then kill the bugs before they can attack.

Exercise for health. A healthy lifestyle is one of the simplest ways to protect yourself from the flu and other infections. Exercise and eat a balanced diet, and your immune system could pack the punch of George Foreman.

Save yourself with selenium. Found in meat, wheat, rice, and other grains, selenium is part of an antioxidant that helps your body fight off infections. A shortage of selenium could therefore weaken your immune system and lead to a more severe case of the flu. Deficiencies of certain nutrients like selenium may also lead to mutations in flu bugs and other viruses, creating even more harmful germs.

Most people don't have to worry about getting enough selenium. But if you don't eat a balanced diet, or if you have chronic heart or lung disease, you might be at risk. Talk with your doctor about supplements.

Ease out of colds with echinacea. Echinacea could be your ticket out of a cold. Experts agree — the herb can cut the time you spend sick and lessen the severity of your symptoms. If you're taking echinacea extract, the recommended dose is 300 milligrams (mg) three times a day. For whole herb supplements, take 1 to 2 grams three times a day.

Whichever kind you use, start as soon as you feel sniffly and sneezy, and keep taking it for one to two weeks. But be careful — echinacea is good for short-term relief, but not long-term prevention. Using echinacea on a regular basis for too long can actually weaken your immune system.

What is it?

Colds and influenza (flu) are highly contagious viral infections of your respiratory system. A cold is a minor infection that affects your nose and throat. The flu is more serious and can lead to other problems, such as pneumonia.

Symptoms, cold:
- Stuffy and/or runny nose
- Sore throat
- Sneezing
- Coughing

Symptoms, flu:
- Cold symptoms
- Fatigue
- Headache
- Muscle aches
- Fever, chills

Soap up. While washing your hands could be the best way to get those bugs before they get you, don't buy special antibacterial soap to get the job done. Since viruses cause colds and flu, the antibacterial chemical in these soaps will have no effect on them anyway. If you just want to get clean, plain old soap will do — it's the actual motion of washing your hands that gets rid of most bacteria. Besides, antibacterial soap can actually do more harm than good. It's probably killing just as many good bacteria as bad, and creating antibiotic-resistant super bugs in the process.

Say no to mold. A damp home is just not good for your lungs. Mold and mildew may trigger inflammation in your respiratory system, leaving you more vulnerable to colds.

Search out the safest herbs

Taking an herbal remedy for a cold is natural but not always safe. According to recent research, dangerous bacteria and molds taint many favorites, like echinacea, St. John's wort, and kava kava. If you are seriously ill and have a weakened immune system, these herbal stowaways can be especially harmful.

Most of the time, critters hitch a ride on herbs bought in "bulk," like you might find in barrels at a natural food store or organic co-operative. But even capsules of organically grown herbs can contain bacteria, perhaps from natural fertilizers.

The problem — no regulation. Researchers compared herbs to regulated drugs that health authorities inspect, like aspirin and acetaminophen. These over-the-counter medicines were completely free of contaminants.

For most healthy people, the bacteria and molds pose little risk. Still, if you want to avoid them, experts recommend doing your homework and buying only standardized herbal extracts from trusted companies.

The biggest risks are the patches of fungus you can actually see. Not only will they put you in danger of getting more viral infections, but they also weaken your resistance to bronchitis, pneumonia, and allergies. That's enough to make you take on spring-cleaning in spring, summer, fall, and winter.

Tea off on germs. Killing viruses might be as easy as enjoying a cool glass of iced tea on a hot summer day. While researchers haven't tested their theory on animals or humans yet, they believe certain varieties of tea may knock out viruses almost on contact.

Black tea seemed to work better than the green variety, and store-bought iced teas worked just as well as the home-brewed kind.

Inject more power into your flu shot

Your next bout with influenza might be more than an inconvenience — it could be deadly. Although flu season affects everyone, it especially takes its toll on seniors. If you're over 65, your odds of becoming seriously ill — or even dying — from the flu skyrocket.

Getting a flu shot gives you the best protection, and doctors recommend it yearly for anyone over 50. Try to get vaccinated between mid-October and mid-November, although you can do it anytime from September through March. Experts estimate that if everyone got a flu shot as suggested, it would prevent 70 percent of hospitalizations and 80 percent of deaths related to flu.

By taking a few extra steps, you can protect yourself even further. Here's how to get the most out of your flu shot.

Grab some ginseng. A recent study found that taking 100 milligrams of this herbal supplement twice a day for four months enhanced the power of a flu shot. By giving your immune system a boost, ginseng reinforces your body's battle against the flu.

Relax. If you're under a lot of stress, your body won't respond properly to the flu shot. Studies show that chronic stress works against your immune system. So, find ways to deal with your anxieties. Try some light exercise, find someone to talk to about your problems, or just meditate. Maybe even take a stress management class. Remember, reducing your stress might reduce your chances of getting the flu.

Be a cautious traveler. Unlike the United States, countries in the Southern hemisphere suffer their flu season from April to September. In some tropical areas, flu season is year-round. But even if you're not visiting any of these places, others in your tour group or on your plane or cruise ship could infect you. Experts advise getting a flu shot before you travel. If the current vaccine is not yet available, ask your doctor about antiviral medication you can take with you in case you get sick on your trip.

Pop pills the proper way

Strange, but true. Don't tilt your head back when swallowing a pill. Instead, bring your head forward so your chin nearly touches your chest.

With this method, there's no danger of the pill going down the wrong tube and becoming lodged in your windpipe. You're also less likely to gag.

And always take your time. Even if you have several medications and other things to do, stand still, concentrate on what you're doing, and swallow one pill at a time. It might take longer, but it might also save your life.

Improve your odds of staying healthy

All through the winter months, you get cold after cold. Just when you think it's over, you come down with the flu. You feel lousy, you act grumpy, and you think life just isn't fair. Why is it your neighbor, your co-worker, even your spouse never get a sniffle?

It's not necessarily stronger genes, better hygiene, or cleaner living. New research suggests your health might be your own choice — will you be happy and well or cranky and sick?

Choose cheerfulness. Having a negative personality actually puts you at higher risk for colds.

In a yearlong study at a Spanish university, researchers tracked more than 1,000 people and the number of colds they caught. As expected, people under stress suffered more. Those with negative personalities — often called pessimists — were more sensitive to stress, and were nearly three times as likely to catch a cold as positive, optimistic people.

If you tend to be negative, watch positive people in action and study how they react to life. Then, try to practice positive thinking whenever possible. Consider counseling if you just can't seem to break negative patterns. At any age, you can learn new ways to respond to the stress in your life.

Find work that fits. Stress from a job that doesn't match your personality can cause you to be sick more often. Let's say you have a job that allows you to make decisions and you have the self-confidence to make these decisions. Experts claim you're less likely to suffer from infections, like colds and the flu. In other words, if you're prepared mentally to handle the extra stress of more work and more responsibility, you'll save your immune system.

On the other hand, people who tend to blame themselves for mistakes are better off in an occupation that doesn't require much decision-making.

Whether you're looking for a second career or volunteer work, check out books with personality tests that can match you to different occupations. Find work that fits your character traits, and you'll enjoy better health.

Forgive others. Holding a grudge, according to an expert in psychology, has both an emotional and a physical cost.

Charlotte Van Oyen Witvliet, Assistant Professor of Psychology at Hope College in Michigan, recently asked people to think angrily of someone who had hurt them in the past. Almost immediately, their heart rate, blood pressure, and sweating increased — typical signs of stress.

"These unforgiving responses," Witvliet says, "stir up negative emotions, reduce perceived control, and are physically stressful."

But when she asked them to understand and forgive the people who hurt them, stress levels dropped significantly. "People reported higher levels of positive emotion and perceived control, and they experienced less physiological stress."

A lifetime of anger and bitterness can wear away your natural resistance to infection and disease. Even though you can't change the past, Witvliet encourages you to change how you think about it — for the good of your health.

Cooking superstar conquers colds

Give the cold shoulder to congestion, sore throats, and bland food with a clove of garlic. Not only will it zest up your meal, it will boost your immune system — thanks to allicin. This natural compound, released when you crush the cloves, is what gives garlic its

Pluck a pomegranate to cure a cold

People living in the Middle East know what to do when a nasty cold strikes — grab a pomegranate.

On the outside, this fruit looks a bit like old leather. But inside, it's a different story. Cut open a pomegranate and you'll find a bright red, delicious fruit that's high in vitamin C — just what you need for a cold.

Start slurping sweet pomegranate juice at the first sign of a cold and you'll start treating your sore throat, cough, and congestion. It's also a delicious way to keep up your fluids.

Vitamin C is quite a wonder. Besides helping your cold, it's important for sharp vision and healthy skin and bones. You need it for vigorous cell growth and reproduction. And if that's not enough from one little vitamin, researchers think it can help protect you from arthritis, cancer, heart disease, memory loss, respiratory distress syndrome, liver disease, diabetes, and Parkinson's disease.

flavor and aroma. Allicin works to fight colds, the flu, and other infections by breaking down into smaller chemicals called sulfur compounds. They jump-start your immune system, helping your body get rid of harmful toxins and microorganisms naturally.

More importantly, allicin acts like an antibiotic. It's been called "Russian penicillin" for its ability to help the body fight off infections, particularly respiratory and digestive infections. Military studies from World War II showed that soldiers who ate the most garlic had the fewest cases of dysentery.

You name it and the allicin in garlic seems to kill it — bacteria, molds, viruses, yeasts, and other parasites. Some of its victims include *H. pylori,* the bug behind stomach ulcers, as well as *Salmonella* and *E. coli*.

Mincing fresh garlic seems to be the best way to get all of the benefits of allicin. Experts recommend eating from one-half to three cloves a day. You can also try garlic powder or supplements. Whatever type you consider, talk with your doctor if you're taking blood-thinning medication like warfarin.

5 ways to fight superbugs

Antibiotic resistance is becoming a major problem in health care. The Centers for Disease Control and Prevention (CDC) estimate that up to half of the 235 million doses of antibiotics taken each year are probably unnecessary. This allows bacteria to develop new strains that can resist these drugs.

You can help fight these powerful superbugs by following a few guidelines:

➥ Don't ask your doctor to prescribe an antibiotic for a cold or the flu. Antibiotics are useless against viral infections. Many doctors say they prescribe an antibiotic because their patients expect or request it.

- If your doctor prescribes an antibiotic, ask questions. Make sure it is necessary for you to take that drug.

- Follow directions given by your doctor or pharmacist exactly. Take your medicine at the proper time, and finish the entire prescription. Don't stop taking it just because you feel better. You may not have killed all the bacteria.

- Always wash your hands thoroughly and handle food properly to prevent spreading bacteria in the first place.

- Never save medication to give to someone else later.

Folk Remedy

Chicken soup as a cold remedy goes back long before your grandmother — or even your great-grandmother. In 60 A.D., an army surgeon to Roman emperor Nero wrote of it in his journals. A thousand years later, another physician stated, "Chicken soup ... is recommended as an excellent food as well as medication."

CONSTIPATION

Expert help for constipation

It's time to make some changes if constipation is your constant companion. Irregularity can make you uncomfortable, grumpy, and out of sorts, but chronic constipation can lead to painful hemorrhoids, diverticulosis, and certain kinds of cancer.

But don't let that scare you into taking a laxative at the first sign of constipation. You can become dependent on these medications, and they may lose their effectiveness if you use them often. Over-use can cause cramping, diarrhea, and dehydration. Those containing magnesium can have even more serious side effects, like breathing difficulties, irregular heartbeat, and even coma.

The best way to control constipation is to do it nature's way. Here's how you can get relief:

Eat more roughage. "It is definitely wise," says Dr. Ruth Peters, research scientist and professor of preventive medicine at the University of Southern California, "for

What is it?

If you're constipated, you have infrequent bowel movements, and your stool is often hard and difficult to pass. Some people naturally have fewer bowel movements than others — therefore, what is infrequent for one person might be perfectly normal for someone else. If you have fewer than two bowel movements a week, however, you are probably constipated.

Symptoms:
- ✧ Infrequent bowel movements
- ✧ Hard, dry stool that is difficult to pass
- ✧ Straining during bowel movements
- ✧ Abdominal bloating and discomfort

67

anyone with constipation to add fiber to their diet." Eating fruits, vegetables, and whole grains — all rich in fiber — adds bulk to your stool and helps it move more quickly through your digestive tract.

Since the 1970s, experts have recommended fiber not only for constipation but for reducing the risk of colon cancer as well. Recently, there has been a great deal of debate on this subject, since a number of studies have not found that fiber lowers this risk.

"In my own case-control study on colon cancer, we did not find a strong link between dietary fiber consumption and the risk of colon cancer," says Peters. "But in an earlier study, we did observe a strong link between severe hemorrhoids and the risk of anal cancer — and fiber is a recommended treatment for hemorrhoids."

Dr. Robert Goodlad of the Imperial Cancer Research Fund in London, who has most strongly pointed out the weaknesses of the link to colon cancer, says, "I still advocate eating plenty of fiber-rich foods and would favor fruits and vegetables over cereal fiber."

Yet, Goodlad recommends avoiding fiber supplements, which are made from the outer shells of seeds. They may be lacking what you need for protection if it turns out that something other than fiber in a high-fiber diet protects you from colon cancer.

If you haven't been eating a lot of fiber, add it gradually so your system can adjust to it. Otherwise, you might experience diarrhea, cramps, or bloating. Try to keep your fiber intake within the recommended range of 20 to 35 grams a day. Some research suggests that excessive fiber, especially from supplements, could even increase, rather than decrease, your risk of colon cancer.

Move your body to move your bowels. You may not think about exercise as a solution to your constipation problem, but regular physical activity — as simple as a brisk daily walk around the block — can help your digestive system work more smoothly.

Wash away waste. "Drinking lots of water every day is also a good idea," says Peters. Liquids keep your stool soft, which helps it move easily through your digestive tract. Drink at least six 8-ounce glasses each day, especially when eating more fiber, to avoid an intestinal blockage.

Be aware that coffee and tea are diuretics, causing your body to lose water. And milk can cause constipation in some people.

Keep regular bathroom habits. Setting aside time after breakfast or dinner for normal bowel movements will make it easier to stay regular. Listen to your body and make time for the toilet whenever nature calls.

You may occasionally need a laxative, even if you follow these practices. A mild one, from time to time, shouldn't do any harm. But if you need them regularly, or for more than seven days in a row, see your doctor to rule out a blockage or other serious condition.

Herbal relief for irregularity

Over 4 million people say they feel constipated most of the time. It's no wonder Americans alone spend almost $750 million dollars a year on laxatives. Before you spend any more money, get the facts. All laxatives promise the same thing, but not all of them can deliver.

The next time you feel constipated, check out our tables of proven, natural remedies. These herbal laxatives should be available at your local herb shop or health food store as teas, capsules, pills, or powders. You can also find many of them in over-the-counter medications. Just look for their names — such as senna, psyllium, or castor oil — on the product's label under "active ingredients."

The tables on pages 70-71 are divided into two main types of laxatives — the kind that act like fiber and bulk up your stool and

Bulk Producers

Benefits:

- Known as the safest
- Light to moderate effects
- Bulk up and soften stool
- Make for easier and faster passage through your system

Warnings:

- Talk with your doctor before using these if you're diabetic, pregnant, or taking any medication
- Drink lots of water and other fluids while using them

Herbal ingredient	What you might find at the store	Instructions for use of pure herbal ingredient
Flax	Capsule, oil, or seeds	1 tablespoon of seed (whole or crushed) with a half cup of liquid, two to three times a day
Glucomannan	Capsule	Follow directions on package
Psyllium	Seeds or powdered husks	2 heaping teaspoons of seeds, or 1 teaspoon of husks, mixed in a glass of liquid, followed by more liquid

Stimulants

Benefits:

- ↦ Moderate to powerful effects

- ↦ Activate the smooth muscles of your intestines

- ↦ Provide relief in as little as two hours

Warnings:

- ↦ Unsafe for more than 10 days because they can damage your bowels and make you dependent on laxatives

- ↦ Can cause cramps, diarrhea, dehydration, and loss of electrolytes, like potassium

Herbal ingredient	What you might find at the store	Instructions for use of pure herbal ingredient
Cascara sagrada	Powder, liquid, tablet, or capsule	1/2 teaspoon powdered bark per cup of water, taken before bed and/or in the morning
Castor oil	Capsule, liquid, or oil	3 teaspoons to 4 table-spoons, taken during the day (not at bedtime)
Chinese rhubarb	Powder or liquid	1/2 to 2 teaspoons of powder added to a cup of water, twice a day
Fo-ti	Drops, capsule, powder, liquid, or tablet	Follow directions on package
Senna	Powder, capsule, or liquid	1/2 to 1 teaspoon to a cup of water, once a day

the kind that get the muscles of your digestive tract to push things along. Not every effective laxative is on this list. Some, like dandelion root, chicory, and elderflower, are safe and mild alternatives, but they might not get the job done as quickly and smoothly.

All of the herbal laxatives listed in these charts can cause uncomfortable and serious side effects. Before you self-medicate with one of these herbs, remember — natural does not necessarily mean gentle. Read labels, including any warnings, and follow the directions carefully.

The best way to beat constipation is to eat more vegetables, fruits, whole grains, and legumes and get regular exercise. If these lifestyle changes don't work, talk with your doctor. Severe constipation could be a sign of something more serious, like a blocked bowel. In most cases, your doctor will be able to recommend one of these time-honored herbal laxatives.

How to choose a fiber-rich cereal

When you're looking for relief from constipation, check out your pantry. The information printed on a box of cereal will tell you just what you need to know to fix the problem — naturally.

Understand labels. A cereal high in insoluble bran fiber helps the food you eat move quickly through your digestive system. Not only is this a natural solution to irregularity, it may even help prevent diverticulosis and some cancers.

The name on the front of the cereal box may be misleading, so you'll need to read more to find out what's really inside. The nutrition information on the side panel will tell you that Kellogg's Complete Wheat Bran, for example, has only 4 grams of insoluble fiber per serving. Post's 100% Bran contains about 7 grams. Yet, you'll find a whopping 12 grams in a similar-sized serving of Fiber One from General Mills.

The more sugar in a cereal, the less room for fiber. Check the labels even on cereals designed to attract grown-ups — like multi-grain Smart Start and Sunrise, made from organic grains. Ounce for ounce, these contain more sugar than Frosted Mini-Wheats.

Don't assume all varieties of one brand are the same, either. A serving of regular Cheerios contains 3 grams of fiber and 1 gram of sugar. But you'll get only 1 gram of fiber and 13 grams — that's over three teaspoons — of sugar in the same amount of Apple Cinnamon Cheerios.

Some cereals, like Cocoa Puffs, don't even have fiber listed. That's because it doesn't contain any fiber, and by law, the manufacturer doesn't have to list it. You may see the words "Not a significant source of dietary fiber" in smaller print.

Consider the other nutrients. Bran is just the fibrous outer shell of the grain. For the most nutritious cereal, choose one that is made from the whole grain. Read the labels to see what other nutrients are offered, but don't give up fiber for extra vitamins and minerals. You can easily get those with a daily supplement.

Some cereals have vitamins and minerals sprayed on the outside. To get the benefits of these nutrients, swallow all the milk you pour over your cereal. Don't leave them dissolved in the milk at the bottom of your bowl.

Munch with more crunch. Raisin bran cereal helps keep you regular since both the bran and the raisins have fiber. Some people find it doesn't stay crisp because the moisture in the raisins softens the flakes. To keep the crunch, why not buy a plain high-fiber bran cereal and add the raisins to your bowl separately?

The experts recommend eating 20 to 35 grams of fiber a day. If you haven't been eating that much, add extra amounts gradually to avoid unpleasant side effects, like diarrhea, gas, and bloating. You may want to mix high-fiber cereal with a low-fiber favorite for a while. This way your digestive system can adjust gradually to the extra fiber, and your taste buds can get used to the different taste. It's also important to drink more liquids to reduce side effects and help the fiber do its job.

'Innocent' culprits can cause constipation

You're getting regular exercise, eating lots of fiber, and drinking plenty of water. So why are you still having trouble with constipation? Perhaps one of these little-known causes is to blame.

Iron. If you take a daily multi-vitamin, choose one without iron. Not only is this mineral a main cause of constipation, it may also increase your risk of colorectal cancer. If you are a woman who has reached menopause, or a man, you probably don't need the extra iron.

Calcium. If you take calcium carbonate supplements, try taking them in two smaller doses rather than one large one, and take them with meals. They'll be less likely to cause constipation, and your body will absorb the calcium better, too.

Travel. When you're away from home, don't be tempted to live on burgers and fries. Most fast food restaurants offer several healthy choices. Eating lots of fruits, vegetables, and grains — plus drinking plenty of water — will keep constipation at bay.

It's also difficult to stick to your usual bathroom schedule when you travel. Yet, it's important to make time for regular bowel movements and, whenever possible, to honor the urge when nature calls.

And don't forget to exercise. Whether taking care of business or having a relaxing vacation, schedule regular activities, like walking and dancing.

Medications. Pain relievers, antidepressants, tranquilizers, diuretics, and antacids containing aluminum or calcium are a few of the drugs that can cause constipation. Ask your doctor or pharmacist if something you are taking could be responsible for your irregularity. Perhaps there's another medication for your condition that doesn't have this side effect.

Health conditions. You may find constipation a concern if you have certain health problems — like lupus, Parkinson's disease, or multiple sclerosis. Ask your doctor for help and follow his advice.

Constipation should not be ignored, but don't create a problem where none exists. Not everybody has a bowel movement every day. Trust your system to find the frequency that is right for you.

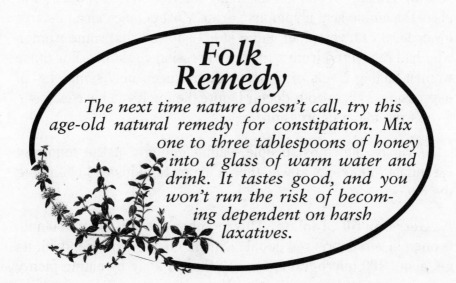

Folk Remedy

The next time nature doesn't call, try this age-old natural remedy for constipation. Mix one to three tablespoons of honey into a glass of warm water and drink. It tastes good, and you won't run the risk of becoming dependent on harsh laxatives.

DEPRESSION

Brighten your mood with food

The food you eat affects how you look. You know that, which is why you avoid those double cheeseburgers and chocolate shakes. But being thin isn't everything. In pursuing a slim body, you may be sacrificing a healthy mind. Your brain, which regulates your moods and processes an astounding amount of information every second, needs a good source of power. What you eat can either make it run smoothly or cause it to sputter and break down.

If you are a woman with a history of depression, you may be at risk for a relapse if you cut too many calories. When you diet, levels of the amino acid tryptophan drop. Most people can adjust to a lower level of tryptophan, but a study showed that some women who had recovered from a major depression could not. For those women, falling levels of tryptophan produced new symptoms of depression. Talk to your doctor before dieting if you have ever suffered from major depression.

If you're like most people, eating enough of the following essentials will keep you whistling a happy tune instead of singing the blues.

Get your fill of folate. This member of the B vitamin family is often low in depressed people. Nutritionists recommend adults get about 400 micrograms (mcg) of folate daily by eating plenty of fruits, vegetables, and lentils. Add a one-cup serving of orange juice from frozen concentrate to your breakfast, and you add 109 mcg of folate. Other good sources include spinach, asparagus, and avocado.

Iron out your depression. Pre-menopausal women and people who must take nonsteroidal anti-inflammatory drugs (NSAIDs) are at greater risk for iron-deficiency anemia. If you have very pale skin, are tired a lot, and have trouble concentrating, you might be low in iron. Some women avoid iron-rich meat to cut calories. If you don't eat meat, you must replace missing iron with foods like legumes, fortified cereals, and plenty of green leafy vegetables. And be sure to get lots of vitamin C since this vitamin helps you absorb iron better.

Seek out selenium. It wasn't until the 1950s that researchers figured out selenium is an essential nutrient for humans. Since then, scientists have noticed that people with higher amounts of this trace mineral tend to be more cheerful and confident than people with low amounts. Selenium also has the ability to make you feel more alert and less anxious, especially if your energy levels are low.

What is it?

More than just a blue mood, depression is a mental illness that casts a gloom over every aspect of your life. You can't just "snap out" of depression, but getting the proper treatment and support can help you overcome it.

Symptoms:
- Loss of energy and interest in life
- Change in sleeping and eating habits
- Problems concentrating or making up your mind
- Deep sadness, hopelessness, or anxiety
- Low self-esteem
- Thoughts about death or suicide

But making people smile is only a small part of selenium's job. It also doubles as an antioxidant and appears to protect against cancer, cataracts, heart problems, and arthritis. In the United States, people get most of their selenium from beef, but the levels found in cattle vary based on where you live. If you're lucky enough to live on the Northern Plains, you'll get more selenium than your friends in the south. On average, a hamburger contains about a third of the selenium you need each day, but you can boost your levels with seafood, poultry, mushrooms, sea vegetables, and whole wheat.

Stay away from supplements, though, unless you're careful about how much you take. In high amounts, selenium can be toxic. Experts recommend no more than 400-450 mcg per day.

Don't overlook omega-3s. Just like a machine, your brain needs oil — in the form of omega-3 and omega-6 fatty acids — to run smoothly. Unfortunately, the average diet doesn't usually contain the right balance of these fatty acids. If you eat a typical modern diet, you probably get plenty of omega-6 through corn, soybean, and other oils in processed food. But omega-3 oils, which are just as important, are often missing. In addition, you might be cutting out too much fat in an effort to lose weight.

In her book *The Omega Diet*, Artemis P. Simopoulos, M.D. explains why fat is so important to the brain. "... Your brain is composed primarily of fat, including the neurons, the cells that transmit electrical messages; if you don't eat enough of the right types of fats, you are depriving your brain of a critical nutrient and risk falling prey to depression and other mental disorders."

The best sources of omega-3 are fatty fish like salmon or mackerel, canola oil, flaxseed, walnuts, and green leafy vegetables. Use mayonnaise and salad dressings made with canola oil, and try to eat fish a few times each week. Say "no" to packaged snacks and "yes" to more dark green salads to help restore your fatty acid balance.

Exercise: A winning way to balance your life

Take a hike when you're feeling low, and you may hike up your mood. Research shows that staying physically active improves your mental health as well as your physical health. Not into hiking? No problem. Any exercise will do — even a daily walk around your neighborhood.

Scientists aren't sure why moving your body improves your mood. It may be that it gives you a sense of control, or perhaps it triggers the release of certain hormones that boost your mood. If you work out in a group setting, the social interaction also may help ward off depression. The fact is, exercise does you good. Here are some ways it helps to balance your mood — and your life.

Stimulates your mental well-being. A recent study found that people ages 55 to 75 who were leaner and more physically fit were less likely to be depressed or to report problems with tension, anxiety, and anger. They didn't follow a regular exercise plan either — they may have just been more active in their everyday lives.

May replace antidepressants. Regular exercise may even be as effective as antidepressant drugs. A recent study at Duke University Medical Center divided 150 people with major depression into three groups. One group took antidepressant medication, one group exercised three times a week, and the other group exercised and took medication. After four months, all three groups improved at about the same level.

Improves your sleep. More than half the people who see their doctors about insomnia are found to have a mental disorder, most commonly depression. Insomnia may be both a symptom and a cause of depression — you can't sleep because you're depressed, and the lack of sleep leads to even more severe depression. Taking a daily walk, swim, or bike ride could break this downward cycle.

If you find yourself sleeping way too much, particularly in the winter, you may have seasonal affective disorder (SAD). Exercise also benefits people with SAD, but it may be wise to exercise in the early morning sunlight to help regulate your circadian rhythms. (See *Shed some light on SAD*.)

Oddly enough, doctors sometimes treat depression with sleep deprivation. You probably remember the giddy, giggly feeling you got after staying up all night with friends. Doctors have found that strategy sometimes works with depressed people, although the effect is temporary — usually only lasting one day. But they think it may help jump-start a medical treatment for severe depression. Not getting enough sleep may cause other problems, though, so be sure to talk to your doctor before deliberately limiting your sleep.

Being more active can lift your mood, improve your sleep patterns, and help you achieve a rosier outlook on life without the side effects most prescription drugs can cause. To maintain the positive effects of exercise, though, you have to keep it up. People who stop being physically active as they age are more likely to become depressed. Instead of giving up on exercise altogether, you may have to change your activity — perhaps take up swimming instead of jogging to make it easier on your joints.

Luckily, the mood-lifting effects of exercise work even for former couch potatoes, so it's never too late to start moving and shake off your gloom. Just make sure you check with your doctor before beginning a strenuous exercise program, particularly if you've been inactive most of your life.

Fight depression with new friends

At 87, Clara Strickland decided it was time to move into a "rest home." Her family disagreed, afraid that leaving her home of over 50 years might send Clara into depression. Her daughter asked about former neighbors or church friends, thinking the transition would be easier if Clara joined someone she already knew.

"No," replied Clara. "But, honey, it doesn't take long to make new friends."

Even if Clara doesn't know it, this willingness to build a strong support network of family and friends is the secret to increasing self-confidence and reducing the risk of depression.

Although you may already have good friends and the loving attention of your family, like Clara, you still can benefit by adding new relationships. Research shows that people who are involved with many different groups live longer, in general, than those connected to just two or three. (They get fewer colds, as well.) Depression also triples your risk of death during the year following a heart attack. Even if you are depressed, having a strong social support evens out your odds of survival.

So, check out the suggestions below for ways to bring more people into your life.

Grow closer to neighbors. Get to know the folks next door over a basket of home-grown strawberries. Gardening can provide vigorous exercise, nutritious food, and a good excuse to share. Fresh herbs, vegetables, fruits, or even a bouquet of flowers can really boost the spirit of friendship.

Be a volunteer. Do something for others and you'll feel good about yourself. You'll also meet people with values similar to yours — a good basis for lasting friendships. And did you know those who volunteer tend to live longer than those who don't?

So don't wait. The American Red Cross might need help with a blood drive. Habitat for Humanity could probably use another hammer. Or check with other charities to see what you can do.

Get with a group. Climb out of your rut and learn something new — a proven way to keep your brain active, increase your self-confidence, and help avoid Alzheimer's disease. Sign up for lessons in bridge, tai chi, or perhaps carpentry. Join a choir and you'll soon be singing new songs with new pals. Take part in a stop-smoking class or a weight loss group. Your new friends will encourage your healthier habits.

Reconnect. If you've lost touch with old friends, why not make the effort to find them again. Perhaps you know relatives or mutual acquaintances who can help. Maybe use the Internet to

Get acquainted with body language

Ready for new friends, but shy about talking to strangers? Let your body begin the conversation.

- **Carry yourself with confidence.** Keep your shoulders back and your eyes straight ahead. Shuffling your feet or looking down may attract sympathy, but not new pals.
- **Let friendliness show in your face.** Make eye contact and smile, even if you feel ill at ease. Just going through the motions can trigger a positive emotion. Smiling with your whole face will raise your spirits and invite a friendly response.
- **Say hello with a handshake.** If you are a woman, a firm handshake suggests confidence and openness. If you are a man, however, a gentler handshake may say you are easy to talk to.

Look for honest and sincere friendship in the body language of those you meet.

- **Keep your eye on the eyes.** The upper portion of the face gives you the best feedback about a person's real emotions. During conversation, most people focus on the lips, nose, and cheeks, but the truth is in the eyes.
- **Notice the nose.** When someone you meet is scratching a swollen nose, go slow in believing everything he says. If a lie makes him feel guilty, blood may rush to his nose, releasing histamines that make it swell slightly and itch. These are also symptoms of an allergy, however, so don't judge too quickly.

track them down. Consider attending a reunion to get reacquainted with old classmates.

Join a gym. Even if you exercise alone, you'll get extra oxygen to your brain, lift your mood, and add years to your life. But working out with others can be more fun and offer a good opportunity to meet new people. If aerobics and weight lifting aren't your style, try a walking, dancing, or swimming group.

Don't think, however, that just having people around will ward off depression. In a University of Michigan study, researchers found people who didn't feel they belonged were more likely to be depressed than people who were lonely, didn't have a social support, or had problems getting along with others.

R. A. Williams, an associate professor of nursing and co-author of the study, believes you must work on your relationships if you want to maintain a sense of belonging. "One of the things that happens with depression," he says, "is that people think no one cares and they can hide how depressed they are from people around them."

Let the people in your life know how you feel, and watch for signs of depression in yourself and others. Symptoms include sadness that lasts more than two weeks, feeling worthless or helpless, fatigue, loss of interest in sex or other activities you once enjoyed, weight loss or gain, insomnia or oversleeping, and difficulty concentrating or making decisions.

Shed some light on SAD

"Rise and shine" isn't just an annoying phrase to get you out of bed. It might be solid advice for overcoming Seasonal Affective Disorder (SAD).

With SAD, you feel depressed during the fall and winter months, when there's less natural light. You oversleep, overeat, feel sluggish, and gain weight. When spring and summer come around, though, you're back to normal.

A common strategy for coping with SAD is light therapy. Being exposed to bright light helps trick your brain into thinking it's spring or summer, so your depression goes away. If you've tried light therapy in the past and didn't notice any improvement, it just might be time to — you guessed it — rise and shine.

Make the most of the morning. Recent studies suggest the time you practice light therapy affects the results as much as the brightness of the light or the length of time you're exposed to it. The best time seems to be early morning — or precisely two and a half hours after the midpoint of your sleep. For example, if you usually sleep from 11 p.m. to 7 a.m., the midpoint would be 3 a.m. and your ideal time for light therapy would be 5:30 a.m.

Stay in rhythm. Light therapy works by resetting your body's internal clock, also called circadian rhythm. Your body operates on this 24-hour internal clock that tells you when to sleep or wake up. In the winter, people with SAD usually sleep more than eight hours because their body clock is out of whack. Early morning light therapy fixes the problem by pushing your sleep cycle forward.

Stick with it. Make early morning light therapy a regular part of your winter routine. If you stop, even for a few days, you might be back to the blahs. Here are some tips on getting the most from your treatment.

- Don't stare directly into the light. It's best to shield the light with a screen and glance at it every so often.

- When it comes to light exposure, more time in the bright light means a merrier you. For example, two hours of exposure will help more than one.

- If you can't sit that long, try increasing the brightness of the light. You should get similar results in less time.

- Talk to a mental health specialist before beginning light therapy. She can determine whether you will benefit from this treatment and can also monitor your progress.

Flowers: A natural mood lifter

Which would you choose — a basket of fruits and candies, a bouquet of flowers, or some other gift — to bring a smile to the face of someone you love? Researchers at Rutgers University thought the fruit basket would be the best mood lifter, but they were in for a surprise.

Flowers, it turns out, brought more true smiles — and more hugs and kisses — than the other gifts, according to lead researcher Dr. Jeannette Haviland-Jones.

"Common sense tells us that flowers make us happy," says Haviland-Jones. "Now, science shows that they have strong positive effects on our emotional well being."

Women participating in the study were told they would be given a present, but not what it would be. They were interviewed a few days beforehand to determine their overall mood. As they received the gifts, all of equal value and in similar wrappings, researchers recorded their reactions.

Researchers then followed up a few days afterwards to see what lasting impact, if any, the gifts had. While all the women appreciated their gifts and showed less depression after receiving them, the flowers had the strongest, most lasting effect on happiness. The women reported feeling less depressed, anxious, and agitated, and more satisfied with life. Results were the same for women of all ages.

Researchers noted the women interacted more with family and friends after receiving floral arrangements. They tended to place them where they could share them with others — in foyers, living rooms, and dining rooms.

Perhaps this response from women doesn't surprise you; but men, you may say, are another story. Haviland-Jones doesn't think so. "When it comes to receiving flowers, men and women are on the same playing field," she says, citing a study by Holly Hale, one of her graduate students at Rutgers.

Hale found men equaled women in expressing their delight and increasing their social interactions with researchers who gave them flowers. In fact, men who didn't get flowers while others did showed a more negative response than women in the same situation.

Haviland-Jones, who is doing a follow-up study on the effects of flowers on older people, is impressed by the impact of flowers in people's lives. They can be a healthy and natural way to manage your day-to-day moods and heighten your enjoyment of life, she points out.

"I certainly send more bouquets now than I did before," she says.

Startling news for St. John's wort fans

St. John's wort may not be the miracle antidepressant everyone thinks it is, according to a recent study in the *Journal of the American Medical Association*. It may work only for mild cases of the blues — not full-blown cases of depression. This is surprising news for the millions of people who take supplements made from the flowering weed to relieve symptoms of depression.

The latest study contradicts the findings of almost 30 previous studies, which all reported that St. John's wort battles depression and anxiety. But according to researchers from Vanderbilt University in Nashville, the old studies were flawed and did a poor job of testing the herb.

The Vanderbilt study was the first large-sized, American study ever done on the popular herbal supplement. For eight weeks, the researchers followed 200 people in 11 clinics around the United

States. All the subjects suffered from severe depression that affected their daily lives. To see if St. John's wort could help, scientists gave the herbal supplement to about half the subjects, while the others received a placebo, a harmless substitute.

According to the researchers, St. John's wort failed the test. Although about a quarter of the subjects taking the herb improved, so did 19 percent of those on the placebo. The difference between the two groups was not significant. The researchers concluded St. John's wort is not an effective remedy for depression.

Dr. P. Murali Doraiswamy of Duke University Medical Center disagrees. "One negative study is no big deal in this field," he says. "St. John's wort is most likely a slightly dilute, gentler version of antidepressant drugs, so it makes sense that it might work perhaps for some people but not for as many as a stronger prescription medication."

The Vanderbilt study did not compare the mood-lifting effects of St. John's wort to those of prescription antidepressants. But a new study by the National Institutes of Health will look at the effectiveness of both remedies and is expected to shed more light on just how well this popular herb works.

Doraiswamy agrees you should not self-medicate with St. John's wort if you are severely depressed. Signs of major depression include having a bad mood that doesn't go away or losing interest in your favorite hobbies or activities, along with problems sleeping, eating, and concentrating. If these symptoms last longer than two weeks, you need to see your doctor for proper diagnosis and treatment.

But for mild depression, St. John's wort may be more helpful than doing nothing at all, Doraiswamy says. And if it doesn't help, it could be a sign your mood change is caused by other things, like thyroid problems or nutritional deficiencies, especially if you're older. In that case, he says, you should talk to your doctor.

In the meantime, consider other remedies for life's rainy days besides taking a pill, Doraiswamy suggests. He recommends exercise, a safe dose of sunshine, and an all-around healthy lifestyle.

"There's no evidence that St. John's wort beats these," he concludes.

Herb/drug combos spark double trouble

You may think that taking St. John's wort in addition to your prescription antidepressant will make you feel twice as good. Actually, it could give you a double dose of trouble.

St. John's wort acts like the antidepressants Prozac or Zoloft, drugs classified as selective serotonin reuptake inhibitors. Using these drugs and St. John's wort together can trigger what's called a serotonin syndrome. You might become confused, hot, sweaty, and restless and experience headaches, stomachaches, muscle spasms, or seizures. Serotonin syndromes are especially dangerous for seniors.

Other types of antidepressants, such as monoamine oxidase (MAO) inhibitors or tricyclic antidepressants, also pose possible threats to your health when taken with St. John's wort.

Unfortunately, the risk doesn't stop there. This popular herbal supplement also weakens the power of up to half of all prescription medications, including drugs that fight heart disease and AIDS. This can be harmful because you won't get the full strength of the medication you need — even if you take the proper dose.

Here are some common prescription drugs affected by St. John's wort.

- Digoxin, a heart medication
- Warfarin, a blood-thinner

- Cyclosporine, a drug given to organ transplant patients
- Antibiotics
- Sedatives
- Birth control pills
- Cholesterol-lowering drugs
- Anti-psychotics
- Theophylline, used to treat asthma
- Protease inhibitors, given to AIDS patients

Always let your doctor know you're taking St. John's wort or any other herbal supplements. For example, kava-kava, another anti-anxiety supplement, can also have dangerous effects when taken with certain prescription drugs, such as sedatives or blood-thinning medication.

You don't have to give up on St. John's wort. But remember, just because you can buy it over the counter doesn't mean it's safe. Your best bet is to ask your doctor if it's OK to take St. John's wort with your prescription drugs.

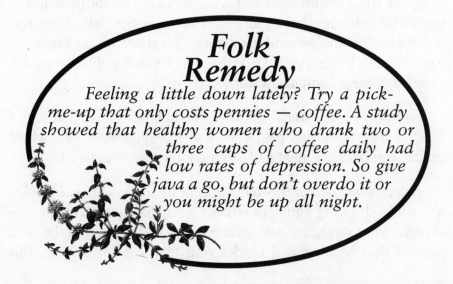

Folk Remedy

Feeling a little down lately? Try a pick-me-up that only costs pennies — coffee. A study showed that healthy women who drank two or three cups of coffee daily had low rates of depression. So give java a go, but don't overdo it or you might be up all night.

DIABETES

Get to the 'heart' of diabetes prevention

Most people with diabetes die from some form of heart disease. In fact, the American Heart Association (AHA) says the relationship between these two conditions is so important, they believe diabetes IS a cardiovascular disease.

The good news is you can take steps to protect yourself — if you know the risk factors and what to do about them.

Get tough on cholesterol. Even if your cholesterol numbers fall within the healthy range, as a diabetic you can't relax. The American Diabetes Association (ADA) suggests you keep your LDL (bad) cholesterol under 100 milligrams per deciliter (mg/dl) and your HDL (good) cholesterol above 45 mg/dl for men and 55 mg/dl for women. These guidelines are tougher than those recommended for the general population. Yet research proves if you work hard to lower your LDL cholesterol, you'll reduce your risk of heart disease complications.

Get those cholesterol numbers in line with exercise and a healthy diet featuring plenty of fruits, vegetables, and whole grains. Cut back on meat and other sources of saturated fat.

A secret weapon in this battle might be tomato juice. In a clinical study, drinking about 17 ounces a day for a month kept cholesterol from oxidizing and attaching to your artery walls — a process that hardens and blocks your arteries. In addition, this amount of tomato juice nearly tripled levels of lycopene, a caro-tenoid proven to guard against heart attacks.

Downsize. Carrying a spare tire in your trunk means you're prepared for an emergency. Carrying a spare tire around your middle, however, means you're at risk for one.

Of course, obesity is a classic and deadly risk factor for both heart disease and stroke. In addition, too much fat in the belly can make your liver produce too much glucose. This will throw off how your body processes sugar and can lead to insulin resistance, an early sign of diabetes. Since 80 percent of type 2 diabetics are overweight, this should alert many people.

Luckily, the solution is simple and helps diabetics in many ways — exercise. You'll lose weight, improve your glycemic control and insulin sensitivity, and lower your blood pressure and cholesterol. A brisk, 30-minute walk each day can do the trick.

Even if you maintain a healthy weight, exercise is still important. A recent study measuring the fitness of men with type 2 diabetes found that unfit men were twice as likely to die from any cause, including heart disease, as fit men. So, being physically fit helped normal weight diabetics just as much as overweight ones.

> ### *What is it?*
> An abnormally high level of sugar in your blood is the hallmark of diabetes mellitus. It occurs when your body can't use sugar as it should, either because your pancreas can't make enough insulin (needed to convert sugar into energy) or the insulin you do have is not effective. There are two types of this disorder. Type 1, also called insulin-dependent diabetes, develops suddenly and usually affects people under 30. Type 2, also known as non-insulin-dependent diabetes mellitus (NIDDM), is much more common. It develops gradually, and most often affects overweight people over 40.
>
> Symptoms:
> - Frequent urination
> - Excessive thirst
> - Increased appetite
> - Unexplained weight loss
> - Blurry vision

Reduce the pressure. If you're diabetic, your risk for high blood pressure doubles. When you have high blood pressure, your heart must work extra hard to pump blood through your body. The strain leads to heart disease. In fact, high blood pressure might cause up to 75 percent of all cardiovascular disease in diabetics.

Again, exercise and the proper diet — low in red meat, saturated fat, and salt; and high in fruits, vegetables, and whole grains — are basic, necessary steps to keep your blood pressure under control.

But to get your blood pressure down to the ADA's new target of 130/85, you might need medication. Another organization, The American Heart Association, thinks ACE (angiotensin converting enzyme) inhibitors are the best choice in blood pressure-lowering drugs. Research shows they not only lower blood pressure, but also cut down on kidney disease.

While ACE inhibitors could be your first choice of medication, they're not for everyone. Even if they help, many times you need more than one medication to get your blood pressure down to a safe level. Beta-blockers and diuretics are among other effective options. Work with your doctor to find what's best for you.

Give up the cigarettes and alcohol. Two easy ways to lower your risk for heart disease — and other health problems — are to quit smoking and cut down on drinking.

Look in unexpected places. Traditional risk factors like the ones listed earlier don't entirely explain why people with diabetes are more at risk for heart disease. The answer might lie in your blood.

Researchers conducting the Atherosclerosis Risk in Communities (ARIC) study found that low levels of a protein called albumin and high levels of several blood clotting substances as well as white blood cells increased the likelihood of heart disease in diabetics. All of these things can indicate inflammation or problems with the cells lining your blood vessels and heart.

Your action plan might be as simple as taking an aspirin a day. The ADA already recommends aspirin for all diabetics because it keeps your blood from clotting. Because aspirin also has anti-inflammatory powers, it might be just the thing to protect diabetics from heart disease. As an added bonus, aspirin also helps guard against diabetic retinopathy, or blindness. Check with your doctor before starting aspirin therapy.

Slash risk of diabetic nerve damage

Nerve damage from diabetes doesn't have to happen to you. A careful diet and exercise program can protect you from the worst of this disease. In fact, the American Diabetes Association says if you can keep your blood sugar in a normal range, you'll cut your risk of developing neuropathy in half.

Ask about lipoic acid. There's a new treatment on the horizon that has researchers working overtime. It's a little-known yet powerful antioxidant called alpha-lipoic acid. Your body makes it to help use energy but it's also found naturally in yeast, spinach, potatoes, broccoli, red meat, and organ meats like liver.

In clinical trials, lipoic acid (LA) improved neuropathy symptoms in diabetics. In addition, as an antioxidant, it fights premature hardening of the arteries, thereby lowering a diabetic's risk of heart disease. It may even help lower your blood sugar.

More studies are underway, but so far, no negative side effects have been reported. At the very least, lipoic acid seems to be a powerful way to fight free-radical damage that leads to disease and aging. You can buy lipoic acid as a supplement but discuss this antioxidant with your doctor before taking it.

Eat to control the disease. Ask your doctor about a diet plan for losing weight and lowering blood sugar, and don't give up if you're serious about avoiding nerve damage.

Restrict your portions and follow the new USDA food pyramid — more whole grains, fruits, and vegetables, and fewer fats and sweets. Choose monounsaturated fats like canola and olive oil for cooking, but use them sparingly. Go easy on meat and dairy products since too much protein puts an additional strain on your already overworked kidneys.

And stick with it. A four-year study of more than 700 middle-aged, overweight diabetics showed very few followed through with a dieting plan. Experts say losing just 5 or 10 percent of your body weight can improve your diabetes. That translates into as little as 10 pounds for a 200-pound person.

Ease into exercise. The Nurses Health Study, which has been following more than 70,000 nurses for many years, says moderate exercise — such as walking an hour every day — can cut your risk of type 2 diabetes in half.

Frank Hu, assistant professor of nutrition at the Harvard School of Public Health and author of the exercise study, says exercise works to help you two ways. "Physical activity often reduces body weight," he says. "We know that being overweight is related to a higher risk of diabetes, so losing weight cuts risk. Secondly, physical activity improves insulin sensitivity, allowing the body to make better use of its own insulin."

As a diabetic, with or without nerve damage, remember you must use caution when you exercise.

- ❧ Neuropathy means taking special care of your feet during exercise. The nerves to your feet are longer than any others in your body and are more vulnerable to damage. Talk to your doctor about swimming, bicycling, rowing, or chair exercises. All these put less stress on your feet.

- ❧ Check your feet before and after exercise, and be sure you don't have any blisters or cuts. Always wear shoes that fit properly — not too tight, not too loose — and comfortable, seamless socks that don't irritate your skin.

↪ Before you begin to exercise, make sure your blood sugar is in a good range. Carry a snack in case it drops too low, and know the warning signs of low blood sugar or hypoglycemia — shaking, anxiety, or extreme sweating.

Watch out for neuropathy

Neuropathy, or nerve damage from continuously high blood sugar, comes in three different forms: sensory, autonomic, and motor.

Sensory neuropathy — often called peripheral neuropathy — means the nerves that carry feeling from various parts of your body to your brain are damaged. At first, you're likely to feel pain and numbness or tingling in your hands and feet. Eventually you're unable to feel heat, cold, or even pain in those body parts. If you have sensory neuropathy, you might step on a tack but never even feel it.

Autonomic neuropathy affects the nerves that control the involuntary functions of your body — particularly relating to your heart, lungs, stomach, intestines, bladder, and sex organs. It may become difficult for you to empty your bladder or digest your food. Men could become impotent.

Motor neuropathy, which is rare in diabetics, damages the nerves that send messages to your muscles. You could have trouble walking or moving your fingers.

See your doctor if you develop any of these problems:
↪ Nausea, vomiting, bloating, constipation, or diarrhea
↪ Dizziness or fainting caused by low blood pressure
↪ Problems with your feet including foot ulcers, or having trouble lifting a foot
↪ Frequent bladder infections
↪ Impotence

⇨ Start with some warm-up exercises and stretching. Throughout your workout, drink water even if you don't feel thirsty. You can become dehydrated before you realize it. When you finish, do some cool-down exercises, and check your blood sugar again.

If your doctor clears you for regular exercise, schedule a workout the way you schedule meals. Exercise is just as important as eating.

Avoid alcohol. Even though alcohol in moderation is fine for most people, it's toxic to your nerves and therefore harmful for diabetics. Just a couple of drinks a week can cause nerve damage. And if you already suffer from neuropathy, alcohol can make your symptoms worse. With stakes so high, why gamble?

Special foods boost blood glucose better

The next time you suffer from a case of low blood sugar (hypoglycemia) don't reach for the candy, soda, or juice. Try glucose tablets and gels instead. They sometimes cost a bit more but they're more effective in raising your blood sugar and are more nutritious.

Hypoglycemia is a common risk if you're diabetic and take insulin. The symptoms include sweating, shaking, tingling lips, fatigue, irritability, and poor coordination. It can happen if you don't eat enough, take too much insulin, or over-exercise. Your blood sugar level drops below 70 milligrams per deciliter (mg/dl), knocking you out, putting you in a coma, or worse.

The best way to pull out of a sugary nosedive is to take glucose products made especially for insulin reactions. These power foods give you the best bang for your buck.

Get help fast. Glucose products are just that — pure glucose — and glucose is the Jesse Owens of the sugar world. In a race to get into your bloodstream, it's the fastest. That's what you want when you're in a fix with low blood sugar. In comparison, candy, honey, and other everyday sources, contain a mix of sugars and sometimes fat. This means they take longer to get into your system and raise your blood sugar. For instance, ordinary table sugar works only half as well as pure glucose. Not to mention, many candies contain enough fat to shoot their calorie count through the roof — up to four times more than a glucose product.

Think of it as medicine. If you're like most people, you have trouble keeping your hands out of that emergency candy stash. Instead of saving it just for a bout of hypoglycemia, you might dig in and snack all the time — an unhealthy habit. Glucose products, however, look more like medication. You'll find it easier to resist your sweet tooth and use them only for emergencies.

Take the right dose. Experts recommend eating a quick 15 grams of carbohydrates when your blood sugar level falls below 70 mg/dl. Give your body another 15-gram dose if you're still hypoglycemic 15 to 20 minutes later.

How can you tell if you're getting that exact dose with a chocolate bar or piece of hard candy? You can't. But glucose gels and tablets come in set doses, so you can be sure of the correct amount of carbohydrates. They vary by product, however, so read all labels carefully.

Don't break the bank. For all of these benefits, you might expect these emergency glucose products to be pricey. On the contrary, they are reasonable, sometimes even inexpensive. Three glucose tablets — enough to ward off a mild hypoglycemic attack — could only run you 35 cents, about the same price as your average pack of gum. See our chart on page 99.

If you still want more traditional remedies for low blood sugar, stick with syrup, honey, non-diet soda, hard candies, crackers, juice, sugar cubes, or gel cake frosting. Your sugar source should be easy to use in case of an emergency and small enough to carry with you wherever you go. Squirrel away supplies in your pocketbook, in your car, and at home.

Whatever you use, always be careful not to give food or glucose products to someone passed out. Instead, either give them a shot of glucagon or take them straight to the emergency room. If you don't have glucagon, on the way to the hospital, try putting some cake decorating gel or glucose gel inside their cheek and rubbing it from the outside until it dissolves.

Extra protein may offer extra protection

Obesity leads to diabetes. Fortunately, the opposite is also true. If you lose weight, you reduce your risk for diabetes. Even modest weight loss can help. According to one study, if you are overweight and lose between 8 and 15 pounds — and keep it off — you're a third less likely to develop diabetes. Lose more, and you cut your risk in half.

Of course, permanent weight loss is hard. The conventional approach involves two basic principles:

- ᴥ Eat a high-carbohydrate, low-fat diet with plenty of fruits, vegetables, and whole grains, while cutting down on meat and other sources of saturated fat.

- ᴥ Burn more calories than you take in. In other words, eat less and exercise more.

Brand	Carbs	Calories	Flavor	Price
BD Glucose Tablets (BD)	5 g/tablet	19	Orange	$1.29/6 tablets (Rite-aid)
Dex4 Glucose Tablets (Can-Am Care)	4 g/tablet	15	Orange, lemon, raspberry, or grape	$4.49/50 tablets (Rite-aid)
Glutose Tablets (Paddock Laboratories)	5 g/tablet	20	Lemon	$3.00/12 tablets (Kroger)
Glutose 45 (Paddock Laboratories)	15 g/dose (3 doses gel per tube)	60	Lemon	$7.99/tube (Rite-aid)
Glutose15 (Paddock Laboratories)	15 g/dose (1 dose gel per tube)	60	Lemon	$7.99/3 tubes (Rite-aid)
Insta-Glucose (ICN Pharmaceuticals, Inc.)	24 g/dose (1 dose gel per tube)	96	Cherry	$11.99/3 tubes (Walgreens)
Monojel Insulin Reaction Gel (Can-Am Care)	10 g/gel packet	46	Orange	$6.99/4 doses (DiabeticExpress.com)
Other store generic brands (Can-Am Care)	4 g/tablet	15	Varies	$5.99/50 tablets (Eckerd)

Now there's another, slightly more controversial strategy that promises results.

Drop pounds with protein. A high-protein diet, like the high-carbohydrate diet, limits fat to 30 percent of your daily calories. However, it doubles the amount of protein while reducing the amount of carbohydrates. You end up with a 40-30-30 carbohydrate-to-protein-to-fat ratio instead of the 55-15-30 percentage recommended by the USDA Food Guide Pyramid.

Dr. Donald K. Layman, a professor of foods and nutrition at the University of Illinois, recently conducted a small study that demonstrated the benefits of a high-protein diet.

In the study, 24 overweight women were fed a 1,700-calorie diet for 10 weeks. Half followed the recommendations of the USDA,

Fetch help for low blood sugar

Get ready to unleash a powerful new weapon in your battle with diabetes. This weapon alerts you when your blood sugar is low — and brings you your slippers.

According to a recent article in the *British Medical Journal,* dogs have displayed odd behavior during their owners' hypoglycemic episodes. Most surprising, the dogs signaled something was wrong even before their owners realized their blood sugar was low. In some cases, dogs have probably saved lives by waking their owners in the night.

How dogs can sense low blood sugar is a mystery. But if you have a dog, pay attention to any strange behavior. You just might be receiving some kind of canine communication.

If you don't have a dog, but have trouble recognizing the signs of hypoglycemia, experience nighttime episodes, and especially if you live alone, consider a pound puppy. Man's best friend might also be your best protection.

while the other half ate the 40-30-30 diet. Both groups lost roughly the same amount of weight (about 16 pounds), but the high-protein group lost more fat and less muscle than the other group. They also lowered their triglycerides, or fat in the blood, and slightly raised their HDL (good) cholesterol.

"The protein diet was twice as effective," Dr. Layman said. "Women eating the lower protein diet were less capable of burning calories at the end of the study as when they started it. We believe this is the effect of more protein, particularly the increased amount of leucine in the diet."

Leucine, an amino acid found in protein, is important for normal growth and metabolism. It also provides fuel for your muscles and helps maintain blood sugar after exercise.

Keep a grip on blood sugar. Of special interest to diabetics or those at risk for diabetes is protein's more favorable effect on glucose, or blood sugar. Many carbohydrates, especially highly refined carbohydrates, cause a major rise in glucose after a meal. Without enough insulin to properly handle the extra glucose, it is absorbed into the body as fat. Protein, on the other hand, doesn't cause this kind of rise, making it a smarter mealtime choice. Some even recommend a bit of protein before bedtime to protect against bouts of nighttime hypoglycemia.

Know the perils of protein. While high-protein diets, like the Atkins Diet, can lead to short-term weight loss, they come with some drawbacks.

- Most people find the diet boring and tough to stick to. Once you go back to eating a normal amount of carbohydrates, your weight comes back, too.

- With all that meat comes a lot of saturated fat, the kind that causes cholesterol build-up in your arteries. You might lose weight, but increase your risk for heart disease, stroke, and cancer.

⤙ A high-protein diet may affect how well your kidneys work and therefore would be dangerous for diabetics with kidney problems.

⤙ While you load up on steak, pork, eggs, and other usual dieting outlaws, you are severely limiting carbohydrates, including fruit, some vegetables, and bread. Your body must look elsewhere for energy. It first uses any carbohydrates you have stored, then it goes after stored protein from your muscles and organs, and then, finally, stored fat.

As in any successful diet, this program tells you to also reduce total calories. Critics of high-protein diets say it's the reduced calories, not the additional protein, that's responsible for the weight loss.

Most sources of health advice, including the American Diabetes Association, favor a balanced, high-carbohydrate, low-fat diet instead. The ADA recommends that no more than 10 to 20 percent of your calories come from protein.

All things considered, be sure you talk to your doctor before going on a high-protein diet.

Fish fights dangerous fats

Go ahead. Order the fish. And don't worry about your blood sugar.

It's no secret fish oil helps lower triglycerides — a major factor in heart disease. That would make fish an important food for diabetics. But for some time, experts were concerned fish oil raised glucose levels. However, when they took another look at more than a dozen studies, following over 800 diabetics, they realized

How much protein is plenty?

Here's an easy way to figure out your protein needs. If you're trying to lose weight, multiply your current weight by 10. That gives you the amount of calories you should eat each day. For example, a 160-pound person trying to lose weight should eat 1600 calories.

To find out the percentage of those calories that the American Diabetes Association says should come from protein, multiply the total calories by 15 percent, or .15. That's 240 calories. Because every gram of protein has 4 calories, divide this number by 4 to see how many grams of protein you need. When you divide 240 by 4, you get 60 grams of protein.

Dr. Layman's recommended diet calls for 30 percent of your calories coming from protein rather than 15 percent. If you simply double the number the ADA recommends, you come up with 120 grams of protein.

Here are a few examples of high-protein foods, including serving size and grams of protein.

	Serving Size	Protein
Chicken breast, roasted, no skin	6 ounces	53 g
Tuna, canned, packed in oil	1 cup	42 g
Soybeans, dry roasted	1/2 cup	34 g
Ground beef patty, lean, broiled	4 ounces	32 g
Salmon, broiled or baked	4 ounces	31 g
Black walnuts, chopped	1 cup	31 g

this just wasn't so. Researchers noted fish oil caused no significant increase in blood glucose.

Fatty fish like salmon, mackerel, trout, tuna, and sardines are high in omega-3 fatty acids — a type of polyunsaturated fat that lowers triglycerides. Remember, that's a kind of fat in your blood stream, which comes from the fats in food you eat, and from excess carbohydrates. A high triglyceride level is a pretty powerful indicator of heart disease risk. Many think fish oil may work by interfering with your liver's ability to change the carbohydrates into triglycerides.

Supplementing with fish oil is one way to get those important omega-3 fatty acids. However, researchers are still working to shed some light on just how much fish oil is most beneficial. In earlier studies, the tested amounts ranged from 3 to 18 grams a day.

Replace some of the red meat in your diet with fish to reduce triglyceride-raising saturated fats. And avoid processed foods, margarine, and baked goods — all loaded with trans fatty acids, another factor in type 2 diabetes. Eating fatty fish several times a week is one smart, healthy way to cut your risk of both diabetes and heart disease.

Diabetics fight back with ancient herb

You've tasted it in curry — now taste this lip-smacking spice again, and see why diabetics are giving fenugreek a closer look.

A bitter-tasting legume, it's been used for thousands of years in Asia, Africa, and parts of Europe to treat a variety of ailments — to settle a gassy stomach, improve appetite, increase a mother's milk production, and soothe inflamed skin. Now Western medicine learns fenugreek may help diabetics in two important ways.

Battle high blood sugar. When people with mild, type 2 diabetes took fenugreek, their blood sugar levels fell significantly. It's important to note that healthy people saw no change, and people with severe diabetes experienced only a slight decrease.

Clamp down on cholesterol. As a diabetic, you're at risk of heart disease and must be especially careful of your cholesterol levels. Research shows taking fenugreek every day can lower total and LDL (bad) cholesterol.

Experts aren't sure exactly how fenugreek lowers blood sugar and cholesterol, but think its soluble fiber and plant steroids, called saponins, could be the answer.

You can buy fenugreek at many natural foods stores, and at markets that specialize in foods from India. Diabetics in this study took about one-half teaspoon (2.5 grams) of fenugreek twice a day for three months to get these health-saving results.

Be sure to talk to your doctor before taking fenugreek if you are on any medication for diabetes. In addition, if you are pregnant, avoid this folk remedy completely. Some cultures use fenugreek to bring on labor.

Beware of hidden diabetes dangers

If you're diabetic, you're already overwhelmed with warnings — don't eat too many carbohydrates, watch the sweets, trim the fat. Unfortunately, while you worry about the major risks, you might be ambushed by some minor danger.

Go easy on the glucosamine. This supplement, used to treat arthritis, can slow down your body's response to insulin, making it harder to control your blood sugar. This condition, called increased insulin resistance, often leads to type 2 diabetes.

Life's pressures may prompt diabetes

If you're dealing with the grief of losing a loved one or planning to move, brace yourself for the possibility of another life-changing event — diabetes.

A Dutch study of over 2,000 middle-aged people found a relationship between major stressful events within the past five years and an increased risk of diabetes.

Researchers suggest experiencing things like the death of a child, serious financial trouble, or the end of a relationship may tamper with your body's ability to regulate certain hormone balances.

Those in the study with the highest number of stressful events were 60 percent more likely to develop diabetes than those with fewer events.

If you're facing traumatic incidents, seek professional help for ways to handle the stress.

You don't have to abandon glucosamine entirely. Just be aware the supplement might have a harmful effect if you have diabetes or are at risk for it. Measure your blood sugar often, and let your doctor know you're taking glucosamine.

Monitor your milk intake. Milk doesn't play by the rules. It has a low glycemic index (GI), which means it won't raise your blood sugar level. But unlike other low GI foods, milk and milk products have a high insulinemic index (II). This means they cause a rise in your insulin level — a potential problem for diabetics. While researchers continue exploring this puzzle, it might be a good idea to talk to your doctor about drinking less milk.

Beware of bitter melon. One of the most widely used natural remedies for diabetes, bitter melon seems to lower blood sugar levels. Although it's in many herbal formulas and generally considered safe, bitter melon does have some drawbacks.

- ✤ It might be toxic for children and cause bleeding and contractions in pregnant women.

- ✤ The fresh fruit contains a mildly toxic chemical in the seeds and rind, so be careful if you handle it.

- ✤ There's no concrete evidence that it works. So far, scientific trials have been both flawed and inconclusive.

- ✤ If it does work, it should lower your blood sugar levels right away. After four weeks of use, if you don't notice any change, stop using it.

- ✤ There is concern it can lower your glucose to dangerous levels if you take it along with other blood sugar-lowering medications. So be sure you tell your doctor you're taking bitter melon.

Folk
Remedy

Just one-fourth to one teaspoon of cinnamon every day could be enough to help control your blood sugar and avoid diabetes. Cinnamon can help your fat cells recognize and respond to insulin better — a process that goes haywire in diabetes. Add cinnamon to your breakfast cereals, beverages, and desserts, and always eat a sensible diet. A sprinkle might slow down this modern-day plague.

DIARRHEA

Secrets to avoiding Montezuma's revenge

You may laugh at some of the colorful names for traveler's diarrhea — Aztec two-step, Delhi belly, and Turkey trots. Vacation calamity, on the other hand, is not all that funny. And that's exactly what you could be calling your next trip if this ailment strikes.

The standard ways to prevent traveler's diarrhea include not drinking the water and avoiding fresh fruits and vegetables. But here are some more tips that will help keep your travels on track, even in a third-world country.

Pack for prevention. If you venture beyond the big cities, you may not find these helpful items. So, pack a good supply before you go.

- Use drinking straws so you won't have to put your mouth directly on a soft drink can, juice bottle, or other container that may be contaminated.

- Wash your hands frequently to avoid the bacteria that cause most traveler's diarrhea. Hand sanitizer or packaged wipes will come in handy when soap and safe water aren't available.

- Habits from home are hard to break. A brightly colored ribbon tied around the faucet may remind you not to drink or brush your teeth with tap water.

Dodge diarrhea at your destination. Once your plane sets down, don't let your excitement make you forget these safe practices.

- Drink only purified, bottled water. Unless you can boil the water to sterilize it yourself, this is your safest choice. However, check the bottle carefully to make sure it's sealed. Refilling bottles with tap water is a common practice in some places.

- Carbonation kills some bacteria, so carbonated water and soft drinks have added protection. Drink them from the original bottles or cans rather than from a glass or other unsealed container.

- Brush your teeth with sterile water. Keep a bottle right by the washbasin as a reminder. If none is available, hot tap water is safer than cold.

- Leave the ice out of your beverages unless you're sure it's made from purified water. Even in mixed drinks, the alcohol is not strong enough to kill bacteria.

- A few alcoholic drinks could have you tossing caution to the wind. Set limits to keep a clear head about safety do's and don'ts.

- Swimming pools may not be adequately chlorinated. Don't go under and don't swallow any of the pool water. Ocean water can be contaminated as well, especially near inhabited areas or sewage pipes.

What is it?

This bowel disorder usually lasts only a day or two and then disappears on its own. If your diarrhea lasts more than 48 hours, you could suffer from dehydration — your body will lose fluids quickly and your bloodstream won't have time to absorb vitamins and minerals from food. See a doctor to avoid complications from dehydration and to rule out food poisoning, infection, intestinal disease, or an allergic reaction to a food or drug.

Symptoms:
- Urgent need to relieve yourself
- Loose, watery stools at least three times in a day
- Cramps and abdominal pain
- Bloating
- Nausea
- Fever

Manage your menu. Use this chart to help you make smart food choices when traveling.

<u>Choose</u>	<u>Avoid</u>
Hot, well-cooked foods	Most cold foods
Processed/packaged foods	Fresh soft cheese
Raw fruits and vegetables washed in safe water and peeled with a clean knife	Undercooked eggs, meats, fish, and poultry; raw seafood
Fresh breads	Raspberries, strawberries, grapes, tomatoes
Most dried foods	Buffet food served at room temperature; salad bars
Purified, sealed bottled water	Unpasteurized milk and butter
Irradiated milk	Tap water, ice made from tap water
Carbonated beverages	Excessive alcohol
Coffee and tea made with boiled water	Food and drink from street vendors

Remarkable OTC relief halts diarrhea

Whether you're home or on vacation, diarrhea can complicate your life. With these easy-to-find, but unusual remedies, you can treat or even prevent that next attack.

Say 'no more' with nicotine. You don't have to be a smoker to take advantage of the nicotine patch. It can also come to your rescue if you're suffering from diarrhea due to colitis. In a recent study, people using the patch were four times more likely to get relief than those wearing a patch without the nicotine. Still, experts stress you should only use the patch after you've tried all other colitis treatments and discussed it with your doctor.

Beat it with bismuth. Packing chewable bismuth subsalicy-late (Pepto-Bismol) tablets when you travel isn't a new idea. What's new is how you can use them. Don't just rely on this over-the-counter wonder to cure your upset stomach — take it to prevent traveler's diarrhea. Experts say if you chew two tablets four times a day during your trip, you could stop Montezuma from having his revenge.

Mix up some minerals. Diarrhea is bad enough on its own, but along with it, you have to worry about one of its most harmful side effects — dehydration. This occurs when your body loses vital fluids. Sometimes drinking water and other clear liquids just isn't enough. Stir a packet of powdered "oral rehydration" mix into bottled water, and you'll get those important minerals called electrolytes back into balance. Look for these convenient packets at your local drugstore.

Give bromelain a go. Its résumé is already impressive — cancer fighter, digestive aid, wound healer — and now you can add diarrhea blocker to the list. Found naturally in pineapples, bromelain is an enzyme that might protect against bacteria called *Escherichia coli*. Food poisoning from *E. coli* is fast becoming one of the more common and dangerous ways to come down with diarrhea. You can get *E. coli* from undercooked meats, as well as unwashed fruits and vegetables.

To prevent it, experts suggest taking 750 to 1,000 milligrams of bromelain a day, divided into four doses. You can find over-the-counter tablets at your local pharmacy or health food store.

Pineapple juice and canned pineapple do not contain active bromelain, so, unfortunately, this is one instance where the whole food is not better than the supplement.

Deal with diarrhea naturally

If it seems like you're spending more time in the bathroom than out of it, find relief right in your pantry. Kill the bacteria that cause diarrhea by mixing three teaspoons of honey with 10 ounces of water. You'll soothe your stomach and banish that bloated, cramped feeling.

Replenish lost fluids and salt with other simple home remedies — like sports drinks, fruit juices, soft drinks, soup, broth, or saltine crackers. More good foods for diarrhea include potatoes, noodles, rice, bananas, applesauce, and boiled vegetables.

These home-grown cures will fight the dehydration that can come with a bout of diarrhea.

- Mix half a teaspoon of honey or corn syrup with a pinch of salt into an 8-ounce glass of orange, apple, or other fruit juice. Then, stir a quarter-teaspoon of baking soda into a separate 8-ounce glass of water. Alternate drinking from both these beverages until they're gone.

- Another folk remedy for diarrhea involves drinking nothing but black tea, with or without honey, until you're symptom-free for at least two hours. Then, eat a couple spoonfuls of yogurt every few hours while continuing to drink tea. This strategy helps stop vomiting as well.

Honey may seem like a "wonder drug" for diarrhea, but that's not all it can fix. Check out these other honey therapies.

- Perfect for minor cuts, burns, and emergency first aid, a little dab of honey can protect you from infection, scarring, and swelling.

- To relieve your sneezing and wheezing from allergies and asthma, try eating a daily tablespoon of locally produced honey. Your immune system will become used to the local pollen in it and won't kick into overdrive.

- If you suffer from insomnia, honey boosts a chemical in your brain that calms you down and helps you sleep.

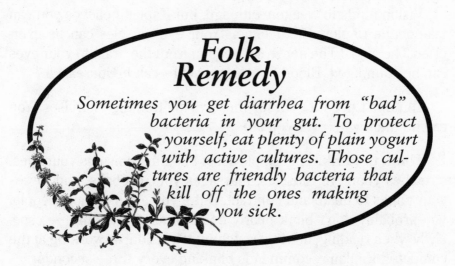

Folk Remedy

Sometimes you get diarrhea from "bad" bacteria in your gut. To protect yourself, eat plenty of plain yogurt with active cultures. Those cultures are friendly bacteria that kill off the ones making you sick.

EYESTRAIN

Sharper eyesight without glasses

To transform a weak body into a muscular one, you must exercise faithfully. If you find that you keep replacing your old glasses with stronger ones, perhaps you should give your eyes a workout as well.

"Just as you can develop your physical fitness," says Dr. Robert-Michael Kaplan, author of *Seeing Without Glasses*, "you can also improve the fitness of your eyes — the way they work together, their stamina, and their interaction with your brain."

Vision tends to weaken with age, but Kaplan believes you can take action to slow the decline. "Your eye muscles can be exercised," he says. "The nerve connection from the brain to your eyes can be stimulated. Blood flow to your eyes can be increased."

You don't need a gym for these vision-training exercises. You can do them wherever you are.

Think to blink. The simple act of blinking moistens your eyes, stretches your eye muscles, massages your eyeballs, and forces your pupils to dilate and contract. But if you are like most people, you probably don't blink nearly as often as you should — especially when reading, driving, watching television, or working at the computer. Kaplan recommends blinking every three seconds.

Practice eye aerobics. Six muscles connect to each of your eyeballs and help them move up and down, side to side, and inward and outward. Here's an exercise that can strengthen them and improve the coordination of your eyes.

Sit with your feet firmly on the floor, hands in your lap or supported on the arms of your chair. With your eyes open or closed, face forward, take a few deep breaths, and relax your neck and shoulders.

Stretch your eyes upward as high as they will comfortably go while you breathe in. Hold your breath for a few moments, and then stretch your eyes downward as low as you can without straining as you breathe out. Do this three times.

Next, stretch your eyes sideways to the right, then up to the right. Then stretch down to the left, up to the left, and down to the right. Remember to stay relaxed as you repeat these exercises.

Rest under the palms. After doing the stretching exercises, make sure you "cool down" just as you would after any workout.

First, warm your palms by rubbing them vigorously together. Lace your fingers together over your forehead with your palms cupped over your eyes, shutting out the light. Rest your eyes in the warm darkness for a few minutes while taking 20 to 50 breaths.

> ### *What is it?*
>
> Eyestrain is a temporary soreness or fatigue of your eye muscles, usually due to overuse. You're likely to develop this condition if you spend a lot of time doing close work without breaks. Poor lighting, glare, and constant refocusing can contribute to eyestrain. Most experts agree eyestrain won't weaken your eyesight or cause permanent eye problems.
>
> Symptoms:
> - Tired eyes
> - Headache
> - Irritated eyes

"When you remove your palms," says Kaplan, "you'll observe that colors are much brighter, you'll see more contrast, and you'll enjoy a wonderful relaxed feeling in your eyes and brow muscles."

This technique, called palming, is also a good way to take a break from watching television or using the computer.

Soak in sunlight. Kaplan says natural light is good for your eyes. He recommends going outside early in the day, before 10:00 a.m., and late in the afternoon, after 4:00 p.m.

To relax your eyes, close them and face the sun, letting it warm your eyelids. Turn your head gently from side to side for about five minutes.

Avoid the brightest time of day and never look directly into the sun. When you can't use natural sunlight, you can substitute the light from an incandescent bulb.

See with both sides of your brain. Your eyes alone can't provide you with sight. In fact, as much as 90 percent of what makes it possible to see may take place in your brain.

The right side of your brain controls the left side of your body — including your left eye — and the left side of your brain controls the right. You need to use both sides to keep your eyes working together.

This exercise, called thumb zapping, is a good way to tell if you are using both sides of your brain. Begin by sitting comfortably in a chair that supports your back. Look steadily at an object five to 20 feet away. Slowly bring your thumb into your line of vision, about 8 inches in front of your face. If you are using your eyes together, you will see two thumbs.

If you see only one thumb, or one is clearer than the other, it means you aren't using your eyes equally. Deep breathing, blinking, and palming your eyes can help you strengthen your whole-brain seeing.

Fine-tune your focus. Your ancient ancestors probably had keen eyesight. As hunters and gatherers, they spent most of their time outside, their eyes darting here and there, always on the alert for food or danger. By constantly refocusing close up, a stone's throw away, and into the far distance, they gave their vision a good workout.

Today, however, you are more likely to spend your days indoors staring at a flat surface, like the television or computer screen. To avoid couch-potato eyes and improve your focus, try these exercises.

- ⤳ Frequently glance away from the screen and quickly bring a distant object into focus.

- ⤳ Hold out your thumb as in the thumb-zapping exercise. Switch your focus from your thumb to a distant object and back to your thumb again.

- ⤳ With neck and shoulders relaxed, practice crossing your eyes. (Don't worry, they won't get stuck.) Focus on your thumb, holding it a few inches in front of your face. Follow it as you bring it close enough to touch your nose. You should feel the muscles pull a little as your eyes turn in.

- ⤳ When driving, frequently shift your focus — from on-coming traffic to the dashboard, to the side mirror, to the rear-view mirror. Look to one side of the road and then the other. Read the license plate of the car in front of you as well as signs at a distance.

In addition to these exercises, Kaplan also has recommendations about nutrition, attitude, and full-body exercise. You can learn more at his Web site <www.beyond2020vision.com>.

Turn on your PC and perk up your vision

If you spend time at the computer — e-mailing your grand-children, tracking down old friends on the Internet, or tracing your family history, sooner or later you may notice problems with your eyes.

Like staring at the road too long when driving, staring at a computer screen can strain your eyes. There's less danger, of course. You won't crash into another computer. But eyestrain can irritate your eyes, blur your vision, and even give you a headache.

Eye doctors call this condition computer vision syndrome, or CVS. Fortunately, it won't do any permanent damage, but here are some tips to avoid the discomfort it causes.

Bat your lashes. The tendency to stare at the computer screen without blinking causes your eyes to dry out. Stick a reminder on your monitor to blink more often. This will lubricate your eyes with naturally soothing tears.

If necessary, you can use lubricating eye drops or a tear substitute for dry or itchy eyes. But talk to your doctor if you need them longer than 72 hours. Dry eyes can be a symptom of Sjögren's syndrome, an immune system disease that needs special care.

Take a break. About every hour, look at something 20 feet or so into the distance. This will give your eyes a helpful rest.

Adjust your screen. Hopefully you have a monitor that tilts, swivels, and has brightness and contrast controls. With these, you can experiment until you find a comfortable position. An adjustable chair also helps you get everything at just the right height. The screen should be 4 to 9 inches below eye level and 20 to 26 inches from your face. Dark letters on a light screen are easiest to read.

Let glasses ease your eyes. If you wear glasses or contacts — especially if you have bifocal or progressive lenses — you may hold your head at an odd angle or lean toward the screen. Talk to your eye doctor about how to adjust your screen for healthier vision. Special computer glasses, too, may help you see better and avoid eyestrain.

Reduce refocusing. If, for example, you are retyping recipes to send to a friend, don't place the original flat on your desk. You have to turn your head and shift and refocus your eyes between the paper and screen. Instead, use a standing document holder, and place it as close to your computer monitor as possible. To avoid eyestrain, the two should be the same distance from your eyes.

Get rid of glare. Move lamps, close window blinds, or use a filter on your screen to reduce glare. Wipe your screen regularly with water and a clean cloth.

Check your meds. Talk to your doctor about any medication you are taking. One research study found medicines were responsible for about two out of three cases of dry eyes and dry mouth in people between 65 and 84 years old.

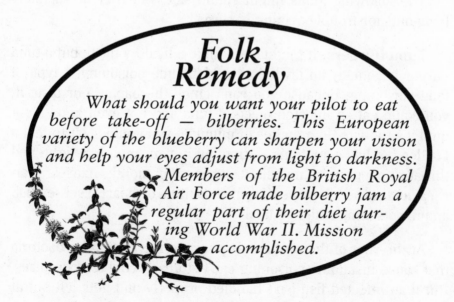

Folk Remedy

What should you want your pilot to eat before take-off — bilberries. This European variety of the blueberry can sharpen your vision and help your eyes adjust from light to darkness. Members of the British Royal Air Force made bilberry jam a regular part of their diet during World War II. Mission accomplished.

FOOD POISONING

Surprising sources of food poisoning

Lounging in the pool on a hot summer day, munching on a healthy tuna burger, taking the kids to a petting zoo — these are all fun and safe activities — or are they? Actually, they're all proven ways to catch one stomach bug or another. You might have already gotten a stomach bug from one of these and not even known it. According to the experts, the symptoms of a 24-hour stomach virus are similar to food poisoning. It's important to know the symptoms of food poisoning and to get medical help if you have them.

The following foods might sound safe, but they are actually hang-outs for trouble-making bacteria.

Tuna burgers. It might sound like a healthy meal, but a tuna burger is actually an invitation to histamine poisoning, a type of food poisoning. Because you can't smell the bacteria or taste it, you could eat an infected piece of tuna and not even know it — until it's too late. In a matter of minutes, you could start to feel a boatload of bad symptoms — tingling in your mouth, a tightened throat, a peppery or metallic taste in your mouth, nausea, diarrhea, and rashes. If you suffer from asthma or heart disease, histamine poisoning could be fatal.

At the root of the problem is poor refrigeration. The bacteria that cause histamine poisoning can't stomach cold temperatures. But if an infected fish isn't handled properly and gets left out at room temperature, these bacteria grow like wildfire. They taint the fish with a chemical called histamine, which brings on the allergy-like food poisoning. Once histamine gets on the fish, nothing can remove it — not even cooking.

You might think the problem is out of your hands, but there are things you can do. In restaurants, be wary of tuna burgers, which seem infected more often than tuna filets and steaks. Canned tuna is also a good choice, since the canning process seems to kill the bacteria.

You also have control over the fish you bring home. By storing it in the coldest space in your refrigerator and eating it within one day of purchase, you could prevent histamine poisoning in your home.

Potatoes. Keep away from green potatoes unless you want to be green around the gills. The tubers could contain glycoalkaloids, natural substances that protect potatoes from fungus and insects. Mostly, these chemicals form in places you wouldn't normally munch on, like the potato stems, sprouts, and leaves. But they can also turn up in the normally delicious and edible tuber — after it gets exposed to light, gets damaged, or goes rotten.

What is it?

Besides nutrients that nourish your body, some foods can contain different types of harmful substances — pesticide, *E. coli* bacteria, even heavy metal. Any of these could make you very sick. You can also get food poisoning from food that is starting to decay. Symptoms usually begin within a few hours, and anyone who ate the same food will probably get sick, too.

Symptoms:
- ↪ Diarrhea
- ↪ Vomiting
- ↪ Fever
- ↪ Chills
- ↪ Abdominal cramps

Once these chemicals start to form, there's no way to get rid of them. Even cooking them in hot grease can't do the trick. Eating glycoalkaloids can make you sick to your stomach or worse, so follow these steps to avoid them:

- ↪ Don't buy or eat any potato with signs of greening, rotting, or physical damage.

121

↝ Purchase older potatoes for long-term storage, since they have thicker skins and can last longer. If you buy new potatoes, eat them as soon as possible.

↝ Keep potatoes in paper bags or in dark, ventilated places, like the bottom of a cupboard. Don't refrigerate them.

↝ Be especially careful with red-skinned potatoes. Green patches could be hiding underneath the skin.

Salad bar veggies. You might be surprised to hear that salad bars account for over 35 percent of all cases of food poisoning. Along with seafood and cheese, produce causes 85 percent of all food poisonings in the United States. To avoid salad bar food poisoning, try making your own salads at home using pre-packaged greens. These are usually already cleaned with an antibacterial agent.

Beans. Just four or five kidney beans could lay you low with a bout of Red Kidney Bean Poisoning, which is much worse than the beans' more famous side effect. Compared with other kinds, kidney beans contain much more of a protein called phytohaemagglutinin. This hard-to-pronounce compound could cause you trouble if you eat undercooked or raw beans. Within hours, you could be battling nausea, vomiting, and diarrhea.

Cooking beans in a crock pot or in a casserole might not even do the trick of getting rid of the protein. And believe it or not, cooking beans at too high a temperature could make them even more harmful. Rest assured, there is a way to cook kidney beans properly and easily. Just soak dry kidney beans in a pot of water for at least five hours. Strain them and then boil the beans in fresh water for 10 minutes.

You can also come into contact with deadly bacteria in several ways that might surprise you.

Petting zoos. If you take your grandkids to a petting zoo, petting farm, or county fair, you have more to worry about than hands that smell like a barnyard. Experts at the Centers for Disease Control (CDC) say you might instead have a dangerous case of *E. coli* poisoning on your hands. They suggest following these steps to protect yourself next time you're on the farm.

- ✤ Wash all hands thoroughly after touching the animals. Help your little ones wash their hands to make sure it gets done right.

- ✤ Keep your hands away from your mouth. That means no eating, drinking, smoking, thumb sucking, or nail biting when you're near the animals. Wait until after you've washed up and gotten away from the animals.

- ✤ Consider not touching them at all. If you're at high risk for *E. coli* — children, elderly folks, and people with chronic illness — touching animals might be too risky, no matter how cute they are.

Acrylic nails. If you are taking care of a loved one who's ill, you might want to give up those long, beautiful acrylic nails. A

Add *E. coli* killers to your food

If you're concerned about harmful *E. coli* turning up in your food, you can do more than worry. Besides cooking meat thoroughly and avoiding unpasteurized juice, you can mix many foods with natural bacteria killers. Adding one tablespoon of pureed prunes to each pound of hamburger meat can kill more than 90 percent of any *E. coli* present. Two to five teaspoons of garlic will do the trick, too.

Other spices known to kill *E. coli* are cinnamon, oregano, cloves, and sage. Season your meat with these for extra flavor and protection, but don't forget to cook meat until the juice runs clear.

recent study found that hospital employees who wore acrylic nails carried dangerous germs on their nails more often than employees with natural nails. Even after they washed their hands, more of the fashion-conscious employees still had the bad bugs on their hands. Their natural-nailed co-workers, on the other hand, scrubbed away most of the bacteria.

Swimming pools. Even if you are parched after swimming 100 laps in the pool, don't drink any of the water. As little as a mouthful of pool water could infect you with a tough microbe called *Cryptosporidium*, which can live up to seven days even in well-treated water. This bug and a host of equally harmful friends sneak into pools because of swimmers' poor hygiene. To prevent this, the CDC recommends the following safety guidelines.

- Wash up after you go to the bathroom and before you get back into the pool.

- Do not swim when you have diarrhea, and don't let the little ones do so either.

- Take the wee ones to the bathroom often — before they start hopping up and down and saying they really need to go. This will cut down on accidents in the pool.

- Change diapers in the bathroom — never at poolside.

- Wash kids head to toe, especially their bottoms, with soap and water before they go anywhere near the pool.

Protect veggies from unwelcome 'guests'

Pork cutlets could have killed Wolfgang Amadeus Mozart. His jealous rival, Antonio Salieri, might have had nothing to do with the famous composer's death. Instead, trichinosis, a food poisoning caused by worms, could have been Mozart's downfall.

Thanks to modern medicine and food preparation, you needn't worry about trichinosis and other meat-borne diseases as much as people did many years ago. Surprisingly, now you have to worry more about catching a bacterial infection from your produce. Fruits and vegetables make great homes for some of the worst guests, like *E. coli*, *Salmonella*, and *Listeria*.

If you're a senior, it's especially important to be careful of these produce poisons. Because of the natural aging process, surgery, or a serious illness, your immune system may not work as well as it once did. You might have been able to brush off a bug in the past, but now the same critter could be life threatening.

Strive for variety. Of course, fear of an infection is no reason to stop eating your fruits and vegetables. Instead, do the opposite — eat more of them. As Christina Stark, Nutrition Specialist at Cornell University, advises, "I would suggest that people focus on getting at least five servings of fruits and vegetables a day from a wide variety of fruits and vegetables. The more variety of fruits and vegetables one consumes, the less likely one will be overexposed to a risk coming from a particular type of produce — that's just common sense."

For instance, some fruits and vegetables are more likely to house dangerous bacteria. Fruits and vegetables that grow close to the ground — like melons, lettuce, carrots, strawberries, and potatoes — are contaminated most often because they come into contact with manure or contaminated soil.

In spite of this, Stark says, "I wouldn't worry about trying to avoid any particular item." Just don't eat one particular fruit or vegetable all the time.

Rinse and repeat. No matter what piece of produce you plan to munch on, Stark suggests following the U.S. government's advice to wash your fruits and vegetables with water and rinse them thoroughly. Water can't guarantee 100 percent victory over bacteria, but it's your best bet. It's also a good idea to wash produce that you plan to slice up, since your knife can spread bacteria from the skin to the insides of fruits and vegetables.

Brush for extra safety. If you want to get even more grime and bacteria off, gently scrub your produce with a vegetable or mushroom brush. For fruits and vegetables with thick skins, like melons, skip the gentle part.

Also, before you wash and scrub them, peel off and toss away the outer leaves of lettuce and other greens. That's where bacteria seem to hide most often.

Handle with care. Just to be safe, follow these latest guidelines from the U.S. Food and Drug Administration (FDA).

- Purchase produce that's free of bruises or damage, or cut these parts out before you eat it.

- Stick fresh produce in the refrigerator as soon as you arrive home from the store.

- Keep sliced fruit or vegetables on ice when you transport them.

- Throw out any sliced produce that hasn't been refrigerated for longer than two hours.

- Wash hands before and after you touch fruits and vegetables.

Sanitize cutting surfaces. Wash your cutting board and utensils with hot, soapy water before and after you use them to cut produce. For the ultimate clean, spray cutting boards and countertops with vinegar followed by a spray of 3 percent hydrogen peroxide. According to researchers at the University of Nebraska, this combination disinfects better than either product by itself.

Shy away from alternatives. You might want to think twice if you're considering using one of those new produce rinses out on the market. Though they claim to remove dirt, pesticides, and even bacteria, the FDA and the Environmental Protection Agency aren't sold on them. Plain old water appears to work just as well.

And as for soap, Stark says that's a no-no, too. "Soap is not approved for use on produce," she says. Since soap isn't food, it makes sense not to eat it. It also goes without saying — keep your produce away from harsher chemicals, like bleach and detergents.

Work wonders with vinegar. One alternative to water that might work is vinegar. Donna Scott, a specialist in food safety at Cornell, says a vinegar bath could kill many of the bacteria on produce, and it's inexpensive and safe to use. To get the best results, soak your produce in vinegar for about 15 minutes. But think twice before soaking fruits with little pores and hairs, like strawberries and peaches. They could absorb some of the vinegar, which can affect their taste.

Enjoy the benefits of fish without the danger

Toxic seafood causes over 4 percent of all traceable cases of food poisoning, according to recent statistics from the U.S. government. At the same time, nutrition experts recommend eating at least two servings of fish a week. That might sound like a recipe for disaster, but it doesn't have to be. Whether you catch your own fish, or reel them in at restaurants or grocery stores, follow these tips, and you'll get the health benefits of fish without becoming a food poisoning statistic.

Run from the raw bar. If you're a big fan of raw oysters and clams, you might not like this advice from the experts — stay away from raw shellfish. Dangerous bacteria and viruses, like

Beware of Charlie the tuna

If you usually eat a tuna sandwich for lunch, you might want to consider changing your menu. A *Consumer Reports* study found that tuna contains enough mercury to pose a risk to some women and children.

Mercury, in large amounts, can cause nerve and brain damage. It's especially dangerous for unborn babies and young children because it can hamper their development.

Whether through factories or natural sources, mercury finds its way into bodies of water — and fish. The bigger the fish, the more mercury it has. That's because the fish got bigger by eating other fish, which also contained mercury. For example, white, albacore tuna has about twice the mercury levels of light tuna, which comes from smaller fish.

Most people don't eat enough fish to be in serious danger of mercury poisoning, but women who are pregnant or nursing and children under 5 years old should be careful.

To be safe, according to the Environmental Protection Agency's guidelines, a 132-pound woman should limit herself to one can of white tuna or two cans of light tuna a week. A 44-pound child should eat only one tuna sandwich a week.

hepatitis, can be hiding in your next bucket of oysters. If you just can't stop shucking, at least follow this one precaution — hold off on antacids before and after your feast. Antacids lower your stomach's acid level, taking away your body's natural defense against *Vibrio vulnificus*, one of the deadliest bacteria in raw oysters and clams. If this culprit sneaks into your body, it can cause nausea, vomiting, diarrhea, and even death.

Shop right. Save the fish for last on your grocery list. If you buy it too early, your fish could become a germ's home away from home. So when you have your cart filled with everything else you need, steer over to the fish counter and follow these tips from *Consumer Reports*.

- ⤷ **Be nosy.** The fish counter has to pass the smell test before you buy anything. If the place reeks like an old fishing boat, pull up anchor and shop at another store. Otherwise, investigate next with your eyes. Check to see if they display their fish on ice. Individual pieces should not be touching each other, and price tags should not be sticking out of a filet or steak. Next, make sure the employees wear gloves when they handle the fish, another important sign of a safe store.

- ⤷ **Pick a doozie.** When the counter passes all of your tests, it's the fish's turn for inspection. A fresh filet or steak will have firm flesh, without any gaps in it. If it's fresh, a fish with its head will have bright eyes and red gills. Avoid any fish with patches of slimy or dried-out flesh, blood spots, or other unappealing marks.

- ⤷ **Take a whiff.** As one last precaution, request to smell your fish of choice when the store employee takes it out of the display. Without sticking your nose smack dab into it, sniff for a strong, unpleasant odor. If you catch one, throw the fish overboard.

- ⤷ **Ice it over.** It's important to keep your fish fresh once you've finally found the catch of the day. Ask the clerk to toss some crushed ice into the bag with your fish, especially on warm days. An easier option — bring your own. Have a cooler of ice or frozen gel packs waiting in your car.

Trim the fat. Anglers beware. The fish you reel in could be full of pollutants, like mercury, dioxin, and PCBs, hiding in the fat. That doesn't mean you should toss them back. To be safe, trim off the fat before you cook them. Also, cook your fish so the fat drips away from them. You might lose some of the healthy fatty acids you've heard so much about, but in the long run, the trade-off is a good one.

Know where to reel them in. An ounce of prevention could lead to 8 ounces of safe-to-eat, delicious filet. One good way to avoid polluted fish is to know which rivers and lakes are full of contaminants and which bodies of water are clean. Then you can plan a toxin-free fishing trip. Contact the Environmental Protection Agency for the latest pollution warnings:

U.S. Environmental Protection Agency
Fish and Wildlife Contamination Program
1200 Pennsylvania Ave., NW (4305)
Washington, DC 20460
<www.epa.gov/ost/fish>

Or get a hold of your state or local gaming officials for up-to-date warnings.

Bring it on home. Whether you netted your fish in a pond or in a supermarket, steer straight home after you pack it on ice. Running an errand or two, on the other hand, will give time for bacteria to build up.

Store it safely. Always place your fish in the coldest spot in your refrigerator. Try putting the fish in a bowl of ice to be extra safe. And if you don't plan to use the fish within a day, skip the refrigerator and go straight to the freezer. Wrapped up carefully, a frozen fish can last from three to six months.

Thaw it out. Speaking of frozen fish, there's a right way and a wrong way to thaw one. Leaving it out on the countertop is a no-no. Instead, place the fish in your refrigerator or your microwave. If you thaw it in the microwave, make sure you cook it immediately afterward.

Wash up. Before and after you touch raw fish, bring on the soap and water to clean your hands.

Savor the flavor without fear. A marinade is a must for a tasty filet, but marinating the fish in the refrigerator is a must if you want it to be safe to eat. Even if the marinade is acid-based — with lemon juice or vinegar — bacteria can grow in the fish if you marinate it at room temperature. In addition, don't baste cooked food with a marinade you used on raw fish, unless you cook it before using it again. When you're finished with the marinade, toss it out.

Finish it just right. Cooking the fish properly is the last step to a safe seafood supper. Just wait until the fish's flesh is opaque, and test it with a fork to see if the flesh flakes off easily. And after you're done, store leftovers back in the refrigerator within two hours.

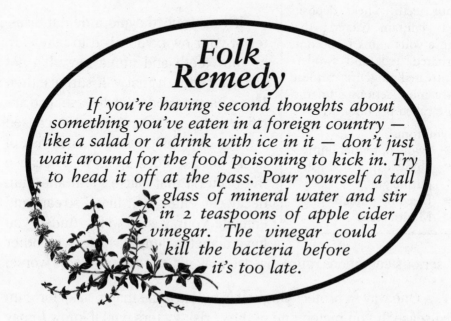

Folk Remedy

If you're having second thoughts about something you've eaten in a foreign country — like a salad or a drink with ice in it — don't just wait around for the food poisoning to kick in. Try to head it off at the pass. Pour yourself a tall glass of mineral water and stir in 2 teaspoons of apple cider vinegar. The vinegar could kill the bacteria before it's too late.

GINGIVITIS

Smart strategies for healthy gums

More than 50 percent of all adults in the United States have swollen gums, or gingivitis, surrounding at least three of their teeth. Almost one-third have periodontal disease, the worst kind of gum problem. Even more frightening— more than a quarter of adults over age 70 have lost all their teeth.

If you want to avoid a dental disaster of your own, you need to take care of your teeth and gums now. It's not just your mouth that will suffer either. If you have periodontal disease, you are twice as likely to have a stroke caused by a blocked blood vessel. Your risk of heart disease goes up as well because the bacteria that cause tooth and gum decay can enter your blood stream and damage your vessel walls. And if you have diabetes, lung disorders, or other serious conditions, gum disease may make your problems worse.

One way to protect yourself is to know the major risks for gum disease. If you match one of these risk factors, you'll know to pay extra attention to your mouth.

What is it?

Gingivitis means, simply, inflamed gums. If you don't remove food and germs with regular brushing and flossing, sticky plaque deposits can form on and between your teeth. These deposits may contain bacteria that cause your gums to become irritated, red, and swollen. Untreated gingivitis can lead to a more serious gum disease called periodontitis.

Symptoms:
- ✧ Swollen, tender gums
- ✧ Shiny, red, or reddish-purple gums
- ✧ Bleeding gums
- ✧ Mouth sores

- ✤ **Family roots.** Up to 30 percent of people could have the genes that make them easy targets for gum disease. Parents could also pass gum disease germs to their children after years of sharing drinking glasses and kisses with them. Short-term contact, according to experts, isn't enough for you to catch the bacteria, so don't worry about catching it from friends or strangers.

- ✤ **Chronic conditions.** Diabetes, rheumatoid arthritis, obesity, and some heart and blood diseases seem to open up a person's mouth to gum problems. For example, the American Dental Association says 95 percent of diabetics have gingivitis compared to about 50 percent of the general population.

- ✤ **Smoking.** According to a recent study, 40 percent of smokers lose all their teeth by the end of their lives. That's because smoking by itself breaks down your gums and your jawbones.

- ✤ **Gender.** About 75 percent of all periodontist office visits are made by women, and it's not because they forget to floss. Women seem to have better dental habits than men, research suggests, but their hormones can affect the health of their gums. Monthly spikes in progesterone levels make some women more prone to gingivitis. Hormonal changes during pregnancy and menopause also raise the risk of periodontal disease.

- ✤ **Medications.** Certain prescription medicines, like some antidepressants and heart medications, can put your mouth at risk. Talk with your doctor about changing to a more smile-friendly medication if you need to.

Whether you're in one of these high-risk groups or not, you don't need wisdom teeth to know that proper oral hygiene is the key to gum disease prevention. So follow these suggestions, and give your mouth something to smile about.

Brush two times. A recent study found you could reduce plaque deposits by 67 percent and gum bleeding by 50 percent — just by dry brushing for one and half minutes before using toothpaste. Start on the inside of your bottom teeth, and then work your way to the inside of the top teeth. Next, hit the front of your teeth and then the flat surfaces of your big back teeth. Make sure to brush your gum line at a 45-degree angle so the bristles scrub underneath your gums.

After dry brushing, add toothpaste and give your teeth another scrub, then brush your tongue for 30 seconds. When you're done, wash your toothbrush thoroughly, and tap it at least five times on the sink so any bacteria-soaked debris falls off.

Gargle frequently. Even if you can't brush after a meal, cut down on mouth bacteria by 30 percent just by rinsing with water. Experts also suggest drinking at least seven glasses of water throughout the day. Water will help your body make saliva, and saliva swishes away bacterial toxins that cause periodontal disease. This is even more important if you're an older adult since your mouth makes less saliva than it used to.

Floss regularly. If you want to take a bite out of gum disease, then you need to floss at least once a day. Wax or unwaxed floss will work fine, just as long as it doesn't shred or break. If your teeth are especially close together, try floss made out of Gore-Tex plastic. And if you have crowns, bridges, or other dental work, check out floss threaders, which act like a needle to thread floss through your dental work. A little toothbrush called a Proxabrush could also help, since it's tiny enough to fit in the nooks and crannies that your bigger brush misses.

Make a date with a dentist. Brushing and flossing can work wonders, but to guarantee a mouth free of gum disease, you need to climb into the dentist's chair at least twice a year. He can scrape away the soft plaque before it becomes calculus — hard deposits of bacteria also called tartar. Next time you pay your dentist a visit, ask him about a Periodontal Screening and Recording (PSR). Previously, only periodontists could give you this test, but now your dentist can, too. That's a good thing, because a PSR tells you how healthy your gums are.

Select your bristles. Experts recommend changing your toothbrush every month; otherwise, it will become a playpen for bacteria. But don't feel you need to buy a fancy toothbrush. Any plain brush with four or five rows of bristles will do. Just make sure it's soft and has the American Dental Association seal of approval. If you have trouble working the brush around those tight spots in your mouth, you may want to go hi-tech. Today's market has toothbrushes straight out of a sci-fi movie — brushes that rotate 4,200 times a minute, use sound waves to blast away bacteria, and even one that lights up when you brush too hard.

Cut back on sugar. The bacteria in your mouth that cause tooth decay and gingivitis feed on simple sugars like those found in candies, sodas, commercial yogurts, and more foods than you'd like to think. By cutting many of these sugars from your diet, you could starve the bad bugs out of your mouth.

Wash away plaque. Not all mouthwashes can do the trick when it comes to preventing gum disease. Ask your dentist about prescription rinses with an ingredient called chlorhexidine. The Listerine you can buy at your supermarket works, too.

Take a break from the daily grind. Stress can put you at risk for gum disease, according to experts. It saps the strength of your immune system, making you more prone to the bacteria that invade your mouth. Stress could also make you grind your teeth at night, a bad habit that takes a toll on your teeth, gums, and jaw bones.

Chew on a healthy diet. People who don't eat enough fruits, vegetables, and low-fat dairy products could be twice as likely to get periodontal disease. The vitamin C and calcium in those foods strengthen your teeth and immune system. So get at least three servings of calcium-rich foods daily, like milk, cheese, and yogurt; and at least five servings of fruits and vegetables like oranges, strawberries, and tomatoes.

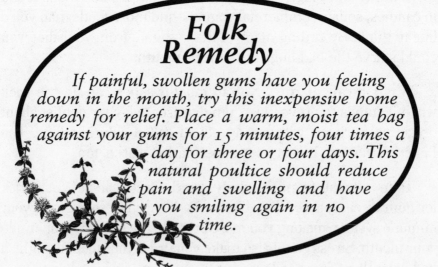

Folk Remedy

If painful, swollen gums have you feeling down in the mouth, try this inexpensive home remedy for relief. Place a warm, moist tea bag against your gums for 15 minutes, four times a day for three or four days. This natural poultice should reduce pain and swelling and have you smiling again in no time.

HEADACHES

Heads-up natural headache remedies

Popping pills every time you get a headache can be a headache in itself. The next time your head throbs and you feel like someone's tying your scalp into a knot, try one of these natural cures. Passed down from generation to generation, these folk remedies are trusty fixes for stress headaches.

Double-team the pain. While soaking in a steamy bath, hold an ice pack on your head. The combination of hot and cold relieves your headache by drawing blood away from your head and narrowing the blood vessels in your scalp.

Wrap it up. Try tying a bandana or handkerchief around your head, just above your brow. This could also reduce the blood flow in your scalp and get rid of the pounding in your head.

Treat your feet. With just one teaspoon of powdered mustard or ginger, you can turn a plastic basin of hot water into a fast headache cure. Just mix the powder into water that's as hot as you can stand. Then pull up your favorite chair, sit back, and let your feet soak for 15 minutes. It's important to cover the basin with a heavy towel to keep the heat in. Keep your eyes closed and your muscles relaxed for the full effect. Your headache should vanish by the time the water cools.

Serve up relief. To win match point against your headache, wrap two tennis balls in the toe of a non-elastic sock. Then lie on your back and wedge the balls behind your neck, one on each side. They'll relax your neck muscles, smoothing away headache-causing tension.

What is it?

Tension headaches are caused by muscle contractions in your neck and head. They are most often associated with stress, exhaustion, or repressed anger.

Changes in the blood vessels in your brain can cause headaches, too. Migraines and cluster headaches are examples. Exercise, certain foods, or a hangover can bring these on.

Other headaches are symptoms of something else, like eyestrain, sinusitis, high blood pressure, or, rarely, a brain tumor. Even overusing headache medications, especially in combination with caffeine, can lead to what's called a rebound headache.

Symptoms:
- ❧ Dull, sharp, or throbbing pain
- ❧ Tightness or pressure

Rub out the tension. Sit in your favorite chair with your eyes closed. Begin massaging your temples and forehead, then work your way down to your neck and shoulders. Breathe slowly and deeply, and focus on relaxing your entire body.

Draw out the pain. To make a handy hot compress, heat up salt in a dry pan until it's warm but not too hot. Pour the salt into a thin dishtowel and bundle it up. For pain in the front of your head, hold the compress to the back of your head and rub. The dry heat from the salt could draw out the ache.

Stop your headache cold. For a frozen compress, hold on to your old socks. Wet them, and seal them in a zip-lock bag in your freezer. Use the whole sock if you want, or cut off the bottom and use just its top.

Help yourself to migraine relief

Migraines mean misery. But it's not just the agonizing pain or nausea that you have to deal with. Often, migraines affect the way you view your entire life.

According to Dr. Richard B. Lipton, a professor at Albert Einstein College of Medicine in Bronx, N.Y., migraine sufferers are three times more likely to be depressed than people without migraine.

"Migraine and depression are strongly linked," Lipton says. "Migraine and depression separately reduce productivity and measurably interfere with quality of life. When the disorders occur together, they produce even greater effects than either disorder alone."

With a condition so potentially devastating, why take a passive approach? Play an active role in treating your migraine. Recently, the U.S. Headache Consortium, a panel of headache experts, came up with a set of guidelines to help migraine sufferers do just that. Here are the 10 steps they recommend.

Understand your headache. Try to figure out when your headaches occur and what might trigger them. It helps to keep a headache diary where you can record all the details surrounding your headache, such as your mood, the food you ate, your sleeping patterns, and anything else you think might be related. Once your doctor diagnoses your problem, make sure you know what the diagnosis means. Don't be afraid to ask questions.

Team up with a sympathetic doctor. Find a doctor who understands headaches and is willing to work with you to find the best treatment.

Share your problems. Tell your doctor all your symptoms. Knowing how often and how seriously they disrupt your life will help him decide on the proper treatment.

Gun down triggers. Your headache diary will help you see what factors may trigger your headaches. Your job is to avoid those triggers. Common headache triggers include cheese, red wine, processed meats, nuts, caffeine, yogurt, and chocolate. New research reveals another potential culprit — wheat. Some people are sensitive to gluten, a protein found in wheat products. When they switch to a gluten-free diet, their headaches disappear.

Discover what works for you. Sometimes over-the-counter medication will get rid of your headache. For example, Excedrin, Advil, and Motrin make products especially for migraines. Even acetaminophen, the active ingredient in Tylenol, might help.

Although acetaminophen had not been considered an effective migraine remedy, a recent study showed it helps some people overcome their sensitivity to light and noise during a migraine. Be careful if you take the blood-thinning medication warfarin, though, because taking the two together might cause internal bleeding.

Have a backup plan. Even the most confident schemers have a Plan B. Ask your doctor to prescribe a "rescue" medication you can take if your usual medication doesn't work. This cuts down on trips to the emergency room. "The greatest advance in migraine management over the last decade was the development of the triptans," Lipton says. You can take triptans in the form of tablets, pills, nasal sprays, and injections.

Don't overdo it. Taking too much medication can make you dependent on it. Overuse can also cause rebound headaches that occur as soon as the medication wears off.

Give your medicine a chance. Try a treatment three times before giving up on it. If, after your third headache, it doesn't relieve the pain, ask your doctor for a new medication.

Stop headaches before they start. If you suffer from migraines several times a week, you may want to ask your doctor about a preventive medication. If you take it regularly, it will reduce the number of headaches you get.

Ditch the drugs. Sometimes, medication isn't the answer. If you're allergic, pregnant, or nursing, drugs can be dangerous. Or maybe you just don't like relying on medicine. Instead of drugs, try alternative therapies like relaxation training, biofeedback, or stress management. They just might do the trick.

Although migraine headaches cannot be cured, they can be effectively managed, Lipton says. Taking charge of your treatment is the best way to ensure you'll find something that works.

"Know your diagnosis. Know yourself," he advises. "Develop a strategy for preventing headache and dealing with it effectively if one develops." Use health care professionals, he adds, as a resource for developing the tools you need.

Something old and new for migraine blues

When it comes to migraines, there's no such thing as a sure remedy. A treatment that works for one person might not work for somebody else. Even your usually trusty medication doesn't always do the job, and you have to turn to an emergency "rescue" medication.

That's why you can never have too many options. Fortunately for migraine sufferers, new remedies might be just around the corner. Here's a preview of two possible fixes of the future as well as a rundown of some tried and true migraine stoppers.

Look on the horizon. The latest research suggests the following unusual treatments may help.

- ⮞ **Lidocaine patch.** The anesthetic drug lidocaine has been tested in cream form — and it works. Soon you might be able to buy a lidocaine patch. Stuck to your forehead, the Band-Aid-like patch releases lidocaine into your head to ease your headache pain. There is currently a lidocaine patch that slowly releases the anti-pain substance over the course of a day, but researchers are working on developing a quick-release patch more suitable for painful migraines.

- ⮞ **Botox injections.** Botulinum toxin A, commonly called Botox, is very dangerous in high doses. In fact, it belongs to the same family of bacteria that cause tetanus. But in small doses, it can be injected to relax your muscles and stop head and neck pain. It's already used as a cosmetic method of smoothing out facial wrinkles. But it may prove just as effective as a headache remedy.

Keep your eyes open for these and other new migraine treatments. A recent discovery that migraine sufferers often have overly sensitive skin during their headaches might open the door to a whole new line of research — and new migraine solutions.

In the meantime, brush up on some of the old stand-bys. They might not be state-of-the-art, but these time-tested remedies have been shown to work.

Try herbs and supplements. If you're looking for a natural way to treat and prevent migraines, sample these supplements.

- **Feverfew.** The most successful of the herbal remedies, feverfew has been a valued migraine fighter since 78 A.D. You can chew on fresh, freeze-dried, or heat-dried leaves to get the benefit of this herb. Or take feverfew in pill form. One 125-milligram (mg) capsule or tablet a day should do. Make sure it's standardized for 0.2 percent parthenolide, the main ingredient that reduces pain and frequency of migraines.

- **Ginger.** Mix some powdered ginger into a glass of water and drink. That daily approach worked for a long-time migraine sufferer in Denmark, who swears ginger soothes the pain and nausea of her headaches. You can also munch on fresh, raw ginger, or cook with it to harness its benefits.

- **Fish oil.** The omega-3 fatty acid you get from fish oil capsules helps stop the inflammation that causes headaches. Fish-oil supplements have also been shown to protect your heart. Eating fatty fish like tuna, salmon, or mackerel gives you a tastier alternative to pills.

Rely on vitamins and minerals. You know you need a certain amount of vitamins and minerals to keep your body running smoothly. But a little more of the following vitamins and minerals may mean the difference between a migraine and no pain.

The truth about your sinus headaches

You constantly suffer from sinus headaches, but over-the-counter (OTC) painkillers don't help at all. If that's the case, consider this — your "sinus" headache could actually be a migraine. That would explain why your OTC medications don't work since migraines usually need much stronger medicine.

To see if you might be one of the millions of migraine sufferers out there, ask yourself three questions. Do your "sinus" headaches happen often? Are your headaches interfering with your daily life? Do your headaches get worse over time? If you answered yes, yes, and no, then your mystery headaches could be migraines. Watch for other symptoms, too, like light sensitivity, pain on one side of your head, nausea, or throbbing pain.

Visit your doctor if these symptoms sound all too familiar. Then you can begin to get the proper treatment for your headaches.

❧ **Vitamin D and calcium.** This dynamic duo has helped women who get migraines along with their period. A study showed that women not only had fewer headaches, they had fewer PMS symptoms, too. The same combination also relieved migraine pain for postmenopausal women. Drink vitamin D-fortified milk for a double dose of protection.

❧ **Magnesium.** A deficiency of this mineral may contribute to migraines. Studies show that large doses of magnesium supplements can lessen the number and the severity of these painful headaches. You can also find magnesium in oatmeal, sweet potatoes, brown rice, broccoli, peas, shrimp, and skim milk.

❧ **Riboflavin.** Taking 400 mg of this B vitamin daily could slash the number of migraines you get in half. It's been shown to relieve headache pain as effectively as aspirin — without any side effects. Get some extra riboflavin into your diet by drinking milk and eating eggs, meat, poultry, fish, and green, leafy vegetables.

Consider behavioral treatments. Maybe taking medication — or even dietary supplements — isn't for you. You might be able to beat migraines with the following approaches suggested by the U.S. Headache Consortium.

- ⬄ **Relaxation training.** All types of relaxation techniques could help you beat your migraines. These include those that teach you to control muscle tension as well as those, like meditation, that involve visualization and mental relaxation.

- ⬄ **Cognitive-behavioral therapy.** A fancy name for stress management, cognitive-behavioral therapy teaches you how to recognize stress and minimize its effect.

- ⬄ **Biofeedback.** Thermal (hand-warming) biofeedback combined with relaxation training and electromyographic (EMG) biofeedback show promise as migraine therapies.

If you're interested in behavioral treatment, talk to your doctor to find out which technique might work best for you.

When a headache hides a serious problem

After staying up until 2 a.m. working on your taxes, your head starts pounding and doesn't stop until you sleep for several hours. Nine out of 10 headaches are like that — uncomfortable, but only temporary.

But sometimes a severe headache strikes unexpectedly or shows up with worrisome symptoms. Get medical help if your headache seems unusual in any way, especially if you are over the age of 55. It could be hiding one of these more serious conditions:

Meningitis
- Stiff neck
- Nausea and vomiting
- Sensitivity to light
- Fever
  Meningitis is a serious infection of the tissues surrounding your brain and spinal cord.

Stroke
- Weakness or inability to move one side of your body
- Confusion
- Drowsiness
  If you have these symptoms, don't delay in getting help.

Brain tumor
- Loss of vision
- Trouble talking
- Nausea or vomiting
- Seizure

Concussion
- Dizziness after a head injury
- Blurred vision or unequal pupil size
- Confusion
- Vomiting

Glaucoma
- Dull pain around your eyes
- An enlarged pupil
- Blurry vision
- Watery eyes

Migraine
- Sensitivity to light or problems seeing
- Nausea or vomiting
- Throbbing pain on one side of head

Sinusitis
- Sinus pressure

- Stuffy nose
- Fever

Altitude sickness
- Vision problems/ hallucinations
- Nausea or vomiting
- Breathing difficulty
- Cough
- Bleeding in retina of eyes
- Weakness
  These symptoms may occur at high altitudes, especially above 10,000 feet. Get medical attention immediately. Your brain may be starting to swell.

If you're past age 50, take notice of headaches that start when you begin to exercise and go away when you stop. This could be a sign of heart disease, even if you have no other symptoms. Be sure to mention it to your doctor.

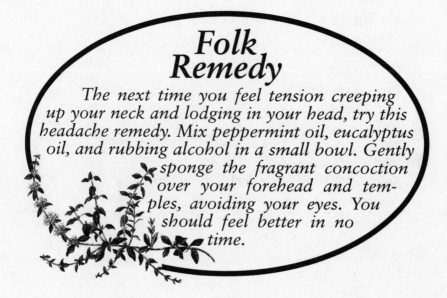

Folk
Remedy

The next time you feel tension creeping up your neck and lodging in your head, try this headache remedy. Mix peppermint oil, eucalyptus oil, and rubbing alcohol in a small bowl. Gently sponge the fragrant concoction over your forehead and temples, avoiding your eyes. You should feel better in no time.

HEARTBURN

Discover truths behind heartburn myths

Almost everyone experiences heartburn once in a while after eating. In some people, their heartburn is frequent or severe enough to cause more serious problems and is considered a disease — gastroesophageal reflux disease or GERD.

You've no doubt heard many myths about heartburn. Read on to separate the facts from these common heartburn myths. The truth might surprise you.

Myth: A high-fat diet is a major cause of heartburn.

Fact: Dr. Roberto Penagini, an Italian researcher, argues that meals high in calories, not necessarily those high in fat, are to blame.

Then again, this doesn't mean you can pig out. Because each gram of fat has nine calories, compared with four calories for a gram of protein or carbohydrate, a high-fat meal is often the same as a high-calorie meal. But if you keep careful track of your calories, you might be able to enjoy a few more fatty foods without suffering the consequences.

> ### What is it?
>
> Acid indigestion or heartburn is the most common symptom of gastroesophageal reflux disease (GERD). It occurs when stomach acid flows back up your esophagus, the tube that carries food to your stomach. You're more likely to have an attack of heartburn after meals or while lying down.
>
> Symptoms:
> - Burning chest pain
> - Pain or pressure in neck and throat
> - Acid or bitter taste in your mouth

147

Myth: You need surgery to correct chronic heartburn.

Fact: A long-term follow-up study recently showed surgery is no more effective than antacid medication. In fact, almost two-thirds of those who had anti-reflux surgery, called fundoplication, still took antacids regularly. People who had surgery were no less likely to get esophageal cancer, a major concern for those with GERD. And, for some unknown reason, they were much more likely to die from heart disease.

Although surgery is still the best option in some cases, such as when medication fails to help, you might want to think twice before undergoing the procedure.

Myth: If you suffer from chronic heartburn, you'll never be able to enjoy chocolate again.

Fact: New evidence indicates a common anti-nausea drug can make your life sweeter. It's called granisetron, and it limits chocolate's effect on acid reflux. University of Michigan researchers discovered that chocolate prompts your intestinal cells to release the chemical serotonin, which relaxes the valve between your stomach and esophagus, allowing acid to creep back up. The anti-nausea medication stops serotonin in its tracks, so the valve remains a one-way door.

For now, if you suffer from GERD, you probably should still avoid chocolate. But keep your eyes open. As research on granisetron and acid reflux continues, this anti-nausea drug might become a widely used heartburn remedy.

Myth: Nighttime heartburn sufferers must sleep sitting up.

Fact: Relief might be as simple as rolling over onto your left side. A study conducted by the Graduate Hospital in Philadelphia found that this position was best to avoid painful bedtime heartburn. On the other hand, sleeping on your right side does the most harm. While sleeping on your back causes acid to slip back into your esophagus more often, the acid takes longer to clear out when you sleep on your right side.

Your best strategy is to train yourself to sleep on your left side. Use a sleeping wedge behind your back to keep yourself in that position, if necessary. Your trips to dreamland won't be interrupted by the nightmare of heartburn.

Myth: All chronic heartburn symptoms are alike.

Fact: Heartburn and GERD have several different symptoms. Not all GERD sufferers experience the usual burning in the chest. Many symptoms actually involve the head and neck. This often makes it difficult to diagnose GERD because the symptoms resemble other conditions, like laryngitis or asthma. These symptoms are becoming so common, especially in older people, that one doctor regularly gives his asthma patients a proton pump inhibitor, a strong acid-blocking medicine.

Unlike traditional heartburn, head and neck symptoms of GERD occur more often when you're upright rather than lying down. They result from a malfunctioning of the valve at the upper end of the esophagus rather than the lower end, near the stomach.

One of the most common symptoms is the feeling of a lump in your throat. Other possible symptoms include a burning sensation in your mouth, neck pain, constant coughing, a feeling that you're choking, trouble swallowing, bad breath, sore throat, and hoarseness.

Halt heartburn. Now that you're hip to these little-known facts, here's a quick rundown of 11 steps you can take to prevent heartburn and GERD.

➣ Lose weight, if you're overweight.

➣ Stop smoking.

➣ Stop or cut down on drinking.

- ✎ Don't wear tight-fitting clothes.

- ✎ Eat smaller meals.

- ✎ Avoid spicy foods and caffeinated beverages.

- ✎ Avoid other common heartburn triggers, such as citrus fruits and juices, chocolate, peppermint, spearmint, garlic, onions, and tomato-based foods.

- ✎ Don't mix food and water. Allow at least an hour between eating and drinking to prevent bloating.

- ✎ Plan to eat at least four hours before going to bed.

- ✎ Don't lie down immediately after eating.

- ✎ Elevate the head of your bed by placing blocks under the bedposts.

Tame acid to protect your teeth

Heartburn, as you know, doesn't harm your heart. And you probably assume it can't hurt your teeth either. But the truth is, that burning acid you taste when you have indigestion may be eating holes in your pearly whites. Dentists call this condition dental erosion. It isn't the same thing as decay, which is caused by bacteria, but the damage can't be reversed in either case.

"One of the most frequent early signs I have found in patients," says Dr. Steven J. Filler of the School of Dentistry, University of Alabama at Birmingham, "has been generalized tooth sensitivity." Unfortunately, he says, people often mask the condition by using a brand of toothpaste for sensitive teeth, and it seems to help. Yet, the erosion of their teeth continues.

"Regular dental checks," says Filler, "are very important and can identify a continuing problem." Your dentist can prescribe a fluoride gel toothpaste that may help slow the progression and make your teeth less sensitive. If you wait until the condition gets really bad, you may end up with teeth that have to be pulled — or at least protected with bonding procedures or crowns.

The most important thing, according to Filler, is to deal with the source of the acid itself. Changing your diet, losing weight, and exercising will help control it, but you may also need help from antacids, like Tums or Rolaids, or H2 blockers, like Tagamet or Zantac.

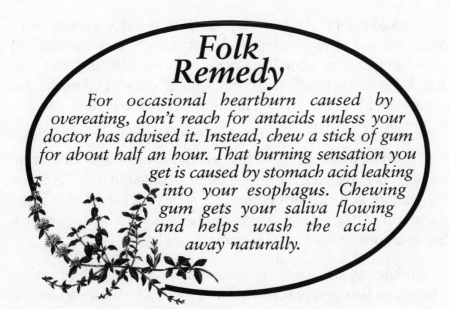

Folk Remedy

For occasional heartburn caused by overeating, don't reach for antacids unless your doctor has advised it. Instead, chew a stick of gum for about half an hour. That burning sensation you get is caused by stomach acid leaking into your esophagus. Chewing gum gets your saliva flowing and helps wash the acid away naturally.

HEART DISEASE

Atherosclerosis

Eat to defeat heart disease

Just as a traffic jam can bring a city to a standstill, gridlock in your blood vessels can do all sorts of damage to your body. If your blood has trouble moving through your arteries, you're at greater risk for a heart attack, stroke, varicose veins, and a host of other diseases. Fortunately, you can improve your circulation naturally with a combination of herbs and food.

Ginkgo biloba. Aspirin can make your blood less sticky and a blood clot and stroke less likely. Unfortunately, aspirin can upset your stomach and sometimes cause internal bleeding. But now you have another option. A supplement called ginkgo biloba, made from a tree that existed in China before the ice age, can also do the job.

Laboratory studies show that ginkgo keeps blood clots from forming, making it a good stroke fighter. Although it works much like aspirin, side effects are rare. (Be sure your preparation is not made with ginkgo seeds, which can be toxic and cause seizures. See ginkgo warning box in *Memory loss* chapter.)

Ginkgo can also relieve symptoms of intermittent claudication, a condition that causes severe pain in your calf muscles when you walk because of poor blood supply to your legs. Many people find they can walk further without pain when they take this supplement. In addition, there are usually few side effects. Take 120 to 160 milligrams (mg) per day with meals for relief.

Horse chestnut. Studies show this seed extract helps people with varicose veins and chronic venous insufficiency, a condition where the valves of your veins don't work properly. Blood has trouble making its way back to your heart so it builds up in your lower legs. Taking horse chestnut seed extract for two weeks can reduce swelling in your calves and ankles as well as relieve other symptoms such as leg pain, itching, and fatigue. Make sure your extract has 100 to 150 mg of escin, the active ingredient in this herb.

Garlic and onions. These two members of the allium family fight poor circulation while adding flavor to your meals. The sulfur compounds in garlic and onions keep your platelets from clumping together and making your blood sticky. Just a clove of garlic a day will help unclog your arteries, but check with your doctor first if you're taking warfarin or other blood-thinning medication. Choose yellow or red onions for the most health benefits. Cook with both garlic and onions instead of salt to help fight high blood pressure, another big risk factor for stroke.

> ### What is it?
> Sometimes called arteriosclerosis or hardening of the arteries, this is the narrowing and thickening of your blood vessels due to a buildup of cholesterol-rich plaque. It's similar to what happens when you continually pour grease down your kitchen sink — the grease eventually hardens and blocks the flow of water. In the same way, plaque blocks your blood flow, increasing your risk of stroke, heart attack — even death. High cholesterol, lack of exercise, smoking, diabetes, and high blood pressure put you at risk for this disease.
>
> Symptoms:
> - No early symptoms
> - Stroke
> - Chest, arm, jaw, or back pain
> - Heart attack

Grape juice. After years of taking grapes apart and examining the pieces, scientists have decided they are healthiest just as they are — whole. Grape seed extract and grape skin extract each, on its own, does little to stop your blood from clotting and blocking your arteries. But when the two substances are combined, the mixture can reduce platelet clumping by 91 percent. And that's why grape juice, made from whole grapes, is a heart-smart choice. Two glasses of purple grape juice a day can rejuvenate your veins and arteries and have you feeling brand new.

Tea. If you have heart disease, you know you run a greater risk of having a stroke. But adding a simple and relaxing habit might change the numbers in your favor. New research shows that drinking black tea can help open up your blood vessels, which might be too narrow because of heart disease.

When study participants drank four cups of tea daily for four weeks, their blood vessels expanded to near normal size. The changes took place within just a few hours of drinking the first cup of tea. Researchers knew caffeine wasn't responsible for the change because people given a caffeine pill didn't have the same results. They thought flavonoids — strong antioxidants found in tea — were likely at work. More studies are needed, but in the meantime, why not try tea instead of coffee? Unlike a new drug with unknown side effects, tea has always been considered safe. In fact, people have been drinking black tea for centuries without any trouble.

Nuts and seeds. Rich in both unsaturated fats and vitamin E, foods like walnuts, sesame seeds, and almonds provide a one-two punch against heart attack, stroke, and other circulation problems.

Unsaturated fats help prevent clots and lower cholesterol, which can clog your arteries and make it harder for your blood to get through. Vitamin E stops LDL, or bad, cholesterol from clinging to your artery walls, decreasing your risk for heart attack or stroke. In one study, women who took vitamin E supplements for more than two years had 41 percent fewer heart attacks. Low levels of this antioxidant vitamin are also associated with diabetes, rheumatoid arthritis, and intermittent claudication.

Other sources of unsaturated fats are fish and olive oil. You can find vitamin E in wheat germ, vegetable oils, and green leafy vegetables.

Fruits and vegetables. These nutritional powerhouses have a lot to offer, including fiber, vitamins, and minerals. Along with vitamin E, the antioxidants beta carotene (which your body turns into vitamin A) and vitamin C help lower your risk for stroke. Vitamin C strengthens your small blood vessels and thins your blood so it flows more smoothly, while vitamin A rejuvenates your tissues and cell lining. Both also boost your immune system and rid your body of toxins.

Eat carrots, plums, tomatoes, and watercress for a healthy dose of these important nutrients. But don't stop there. Asparagus, cantaloupe, pinto beans, beets, and leafy greens provide folic acid, a B vitamin that protects your heart. Many grain products in the United States are now fortified with folic acid because experts estimated that 50,000 fewer Americans would die from heart attacks each year if manufacturers added folic acid to breads and other products.

Flax. Whether in the form of flaxseed oil or flaxseeds, this plant gives you a good amount of alpha-linolenic acid, a type of omega-3 fatty acid that lowers blood pressure and your risk for stroke. This wonder food, once praised by Gandhi, also fights arthritis, heart disease, diabetes, stomach disorders, and even mental problems. It also protects against cancers of the breast, prostate, and colon.

Use flaxseed oil in salad dressings, soups, or sauces, or sprinkle flaxseeds on cereals and salads. Bake with flax flour, or stir in some flaxseeds for crunchy cookies, breads, or muffins. But add flax to your diet slowly — too much, too fast can give you gas if you're not used to it. You'll also find alpha-linolenic acid in walnuts as well as walnut or canola oil.

Beans. By providing plenty of protein without artery-clogging cholesterol and saturated fat, beans and other legumes make wonderful alternatives to meat. If you switch just half of your protein intake from meat to legume sources, you could lower your cholesterol by 10 percent or more. Beans are also high in fiber, which can protect your heart and shrink your stroke risk, and have been shown to lower cholesterol. And when your protein comes from beans and other vegetables instead of always from meat, you improve your chances of avoiding cancer and liver damage.

Dairy doesn't always mean scary

The Milky Way is the name of our galaxy, but to you it may sound more like the road to a heart attack. If you've given up milk, eggs, and dairy products because you're worried about cholesterol, you may want to reconsider. Recent research suggests these items might not be so bad after all. Check out what the experts have to say about some of your favorite "forbidden" foods. It just might bring you back down to Earth.

Make room for more milk. Your mother probably encouraged you to drink milk, and you probably told your children the same thing. But with all the health warnings about eating too much animal fat, you may be second-guessing your mother — and yourself.

Scottish researchers recently found that milk drinkers are no more likely to die of a heart attack or stroke than non-milk drinkers. In fact, drinking two thirds of a cup to nearly three cups of milk a day actually lessened their chances of dying of any cause. One possible theory is that the men who drank milk likely drank it as children, which helped them grow taller. In the Scottish study, non-milk drinkers tended to be shorter than milk drinkers. Long-leggedness in childhood and height in adulthood is associated with a lower risk of dying from coronary problems.

Another explanation is that milk, although high in saturated fat, contains other beneficial things, like calcium, that fight heart disease. Women, especially, need to drink milk for calcium, which protects against osteoporosis. According to an Australian study, older women drink more milk and get more calcium than younger women, although younger women are more concerned about getting enough calcium. But both younger and older women fall short of the ideal daily amount of calcium.

Your best bet is to drink more milk, preferably skim or low-fat milk. That way, you get the good stuff without the fat. Look for high-calcium skim milk for even more protection.

Enjoy eggs. Eggs get a bad rap because of their high cholesterol content, but some critics give them two thumbs sunny side up. Two long-term studies show that eating up to one egg a day does not put you at greater risk for a heart attack or stroke (unless you have diabetes). Eggs do have lots of cholesterol, but like milk, also contribute healthy things — folate and other B vitamins; vitamins A, D, and E; protein; and unsaturated fats. It's possible these substances counteract the damage done by the cholesterol.

So, don't be chicken — eat an egg if you want one. But be careful. The study suggests that people who eat a lot of eggs also eat an unhealthy diet featuring bacon, red meat, whole milk, and few fruits and vegetables. In other words, eggs might be safe, but the rest of your diet might need to change.

Choose less cheese. Americans eat nearly three times as much cheese as they did 30 years ago, according to the Center for Science in the Public Interest (CSPI). Burgers, sandwiches, pizzas, and snacks all come piled with cheese. Sure, that means you're getting lots of calcium — but you're also getting gobs of saturated fat that clog your arteries. In fact, cheese is the number one source of saturated fat, ahead of even beef. It also has lots of cholesterol and sodium, which spell bad news for your heart.

You don't have to cut out cheese completely, but it wouldn't hurt to make a few changes. The CSPI offers several suggestions for making your diet less cheesy. Next time you grill a hamburger or make a sandwich, hold the cheese. A deli ham sandwich without cheese has 6 fewer grams of saturated fat and 105 fewer calories than one with cheese. When you order a pizza, ask for half the normal amount of cheese — and by all means, avoid those stuffed-crust pizzas with cheese oozing from inside the crust.

When you use cheese, try low-fat cheese, or use Parmesan or Romano. These cheeses have just as much fat as others but are more flavorful so you can use less. Limit yourself to no more than 2 ounces of regular cheese a week, and you'll limit your risk for a heart attack.

Remember, cheese and other dairy products provide much-needed calcium — but you'll do your heart a favor if you get your calcium from skim or low-fat milk, low-fat yogurt, and low-fat cheese.

Aspirin: friend or foe?

An aspirin a day keeps heart attacks away. At least that's what you've probably heard about this common little pill. Aspirin actually does help your heart. Salicylic acid, the active ingredient in aspirin, keeps blood cells from clumping together and sticking to the walls of your arteries. This lowers your risk for blood clots and heart attacks.

Aspirin may even help save your life if you do suffer a heart attack. At the first sign of alarm — when you feel chest pain spreading to your jaw, arm, or back — experts recommend dialing 911, then taking 325 milligrams (mg) of aspirin.

But new research suggests aspirin therapy is not for everyone. In fact, for some people, aspirin can be a downright headache — not to mention a health risk.

Here are three reasons to be cautious about aspirin therapy.

High cholesterol may mean low benefit. University of Maryland researchers found aspirin does not work as well for people with high cholesterol. In their study, 56 percent of people with cholesterol levels higher than 220 did not respond to daily aspirin therapy. In contrast, only 24 percent of those with cholesterol levels below 180 showed no response.

This could mean if you have high cholesterol you need to take more than 325 mg of aspirin a day. Or perhaps aspirin is not the best treatment, and you need to find other ways to stop your blood cells from clumping. Even among those with normal cholesterol levels, aspirin only works about 75 percent of the time, the study showed.

Harm might outweigh help. Because aspirin prevents your blood cells from clumping, it also makes it harder for your blood to clot. That means if you're bleeding, it might take longer to stop. British researchers point out that for many people the increased risk of bleeding complications — including hemorrhaging — outweighs the benefit of a lowered risk of heart attack.

To make sure you'll benefit from aspirin therapy, the researchers suggest having your doctor scientifically calculate your heart attack risk using tables from the Framingham heart study. If you have a 1.5 percent risk or greater per year, then take aspirin. Otherwise, it might be more trouble than it's worth.

Stroke risk may soar. Because of the increased risk of bleeding, aspirin may raise your risk for hemorrhagic stroke, the kind caused by a burst blood vessel in or around your brain. A study from Finland found if you have a history of nosebleeds, you might be more at risk for this type of stroke. The danger increases even more if you take aspirin. If you've had nosebleeds within the past five years, think about switching to a pain reliever other than aspirin.

Remember, aspirin usually can help lower your risk for heart attack. But don't just pop an aspirin a day thinking it will do no harm. It might not have any effect at all — or it could cause bleeding problems or even a stroke. Ask your doctor before trying aspirin therapy.

How to fly clear of heart attacks

You may feel like having a heart attack when your plane takes a sudden dip. But in reality, just sitting on the plane might put you at risk if you have atherosclerosis or other heart-related problems.

Experts recently discovered that flying causes a serious drop in the amount of oxygen in your blood, a condition called hypoxia. The root of the problem is the low air pressure in the plane's cabin, which can be the same as standing on an 8,000-foot mountain. At such low pressure, your lungs have trouble filtering oxygen into your bloodstream, and your major organs get as much as 20 percent less oxygen than usual. To try to make up the difference, your heart pumps faster and harder.

For a healthy person, this chain reaction can bring on a headache, tiredness, and other annoying but harmless symptoms. For someone with serious health problems — like blocked arteries, heart disease, or a lung condition — hypoxia could lead to a fainting spell or worse, a heart attack. The cabin's low humidity, plus your anxiety, dehydration, and sitting still for too long, also add to your risk on a flight.

Before you start checking the train schedules, consider these tidbits of advice from the experts. They can help you keep your wings and your health.

Shield your stomach
from aspirin upsets

You and your doctor agree — aspirin is a good choice for you considering your individual risks. The only problem is aspirin upsets your stomach.

First, check the date on your bottle. If you are taking tablets that have been in your medicine cabinet for years, toss them. Over time, aspirin reverts back to salicylic acid, which can be particularly tough on your stomach.

If fresh aspirin doesn't solve the problem, try taking it with food or an antacid like Rolaids or Tums. If these don't calm your tummy, look for an enteric, or coated, aspirin that resists stomach acid and dissolves in your intestines.

Eat, drink, and have no worries. A recent Japanese study found a great way to keep your oxygen levels sky-high while you're high in the sky. Simply make time for a snack and a caffeine-free beverage before you get on the plane.

"Having something to eat and drink is the simplest method of increasing the circulating blood volume for air travelers," notes Dr. Makoto Matsumura of the Heart Institute at Saitama Medical School in Japan. In his study, people with food in their stomachs had almost 50 percent more oxygen flowing to their brains and almost 20 percent more to their other organs. However, don't go overboard before you get on board. The study found that stuffing yourself could have the opposite effect, putting more strain on your heart.

Visit your doctor before liftoff. If you know you have a serious heart condition, talk with your doctor before taking any long flights. For people who fly often and wonder if they're at risk, here's one more excuse to schedule regular checkups with the doctor.

Practice being relaxed. Being nervous about flying only increases your health risks during a flight. So learning a few ways to relax could make your trip not only more pleasant but safer, too. For a start, try this proven deep breathing exercise. Loosen any tie, belt, or other constricting piece of clothing. Then close your eyes. Concentrate on tightening every muscle in your body. When your whole body is tense, relax your muscles, one group at a time, and breathe deeply.

Hold off on the bad stuff. Some people down a few drinks to relax and get over their fear of flying. That's one of the worst things you can do at 30,000 feet. Alcohol makes it doubly hard for your body to get a hold of some oxygen. Plus, it'll make you dehydrated, and dehydration is another major risk factor for airplane health emergencies.

Smoking makes breathing oxygen a hassle, too. Cigarettes wreak havoc with the tiny arteries that take oxygen from your lungs into your bloodstream. If you smoke before you get on a plane, you'll already have hypoxia before liftoff. Bottom line — quit cold turkey, or at least don't light up in the airport.

Impotence: An important clue to your heart's health

They say the way to a man's heart is through his stomach — but women have always suspected it lies a little bit lower. Turns out both areas have important links to the heart as well as to each other.

Read on to discover the relationship between love handles, impotence, and atherosclerosis — and how to firm up your defense against this potentially deadly condition.

Be alert to the impotence-heart disease link. Viagra has given many men a second lease on life. Besides its obvious benefit, the impotence drug has an added bonus of helping doctors discover heart disease in its early stages. Because of Viagra's possible effects on the heart, men often visit a cardiologist to make sure they can safely take the drug.

Dr. Marc R. Pritzker of the Minneapolis Heart Institute Foundation recently tested 50 such men between the ages of 40 and 65 who had trouble getting or maintaining an erection. A whopping 80 percent of them had more than one risk factor for heart disease, including high blood pressure, high cholesterol, smoking, and a sedentary lifestyle. And 40 percent had serious blockages of their heart arteries.

"We now understand that atherosclerosis detected in one set of blood vessels markedly increases the chances of having this form of blood vessel disease in other areas of the body, including the heart, brain, legs and kidneys," Pritzker explains.

"Because the blood vessels that supply the penis are narrower than arteries in other areas of the body, atherosclerosis — the disease process that leads to heart attacks and strokes — may manifest itself as erectile dysfunction before the disease becomes apparent in other arteries."

In other words, impotence can be the first sign of a much bigger problem.

Other studies have reached similar conclusions. A trial by Dr. Kevin Billups of St. Paul, Minnesota, found 60 percent of the 57 impotent men studied had high cholesterol. Of that group, 91 percent also showed signs of arterial disease after experiencing impotence problems.

Of course, just because you have impotence doesn't mean you have atherosclerosis. It could be a side effect of medication, depression, stress, or fatigue, or even a psychological problem.

But Pritzker estimates atherosclerosis is to blame in up to 50 percent of all impotence cases.

"A man having regular sexual activity who experiences a consistent change in erectile function may be demonstrating signs of atherosclerosis where arteries become clogged and the heart muscle does not receive enough blood," he says.

"As we become more thorough in our questioning of patients, it is not uncommon to hear that erectile dysfunction preceded the onset of heart disease by a year or more. Thus erectile dysfunction may be an early warning sign of the potential for heart problems."

Kick irritability with emotional support

Kicking the habit is a good way to protect your arteries, not to mention your love life. But becoming ill-tempered after you smoke your last cigarette won't win you any points in the romance department.

It's natural to feel an emotional response as your body adjusts to the physical withdrawal of nicotine. In a way, it's like grieving the loss of a friend. You just need to learn how to handle it.

Talk to your partner about what you are feeling, and ask for her support. She can help redirect your focus to the benefits you're gaining by quitting, including increased energy and stamina — a real boon in the bedroom.

On the other hand, if your grumpiness doesn't let up, it can put a burden on your relationship. In that case, you may want to join a support group like Nicotine Anonymous. Learning how others deal with irritability might give you clues to the quickest way back to your good-natured personality.

If you're experiencing trouble with erections, you may want to schedule an appointment with a cardiologist and have him screen you for coronary artery disease.

Trim your belly to trim your risk. Before you buy a bigger pair of pants, remember your risk of impotence expands along with your waistline.

Harvard professor Eric B. Rimm recently led a study that determined waist size had a big impact on erectile dysfunction. For example, a man with a 42-inch waist was nearly twice as likely to experience impotence as a man with a 32-inch waist. Rimm and colleagues also found men who exercised 30 minutes a day were 41 percent less likely to be impotent than those who engaged in the least amount of exercise.

These results make sense, considering obesity and a sedentary lifestyle are also risk factors for atherosclerosis. You should begin to see a definite link — a big belly is a risk factor for impotence, which might be a sign of atherosclerosis, which might be caused by a big belly.

If that sounds too confusing, just remember that the risk factors for impotence and atherosclerosis are the same.

Prevent two problems with one effort. Because of the close relationship between impotence and atherosclerosis, the steps you take to prevent one also help you guard against the other.

Here are a few simple, healthy lifestyle changes you can make to combat both impotence and atherosclerosis.

- ◈ **Exercise.** Even if you start late in life, exercise is the most effective way to lower your risk for impotence. So get moving.

- ◈ **Eat a healthy diet.** Cut down on meat, saturated fat, and salt, and eat more fruits, vegetables, and whole grains. You'll help keep your weight, blood pressure, and cholesterol under control.

- **Drink moderately.** Rimm's study found that men who had one or two drinks a day cut their risk for impotence by one-third compared to those who drank more often or not at all.

- **Stop smoking.** You'll do wonders for your arteries — and your overall health.

Sometimes, a few changes are all it takes to save your heart and your sex life. According to Pritzker, "The heart disease found in the study participants was treatable, and in many cases the men's erectile dysfunction went away when they quit smoking or got their cholesterol levels under control."

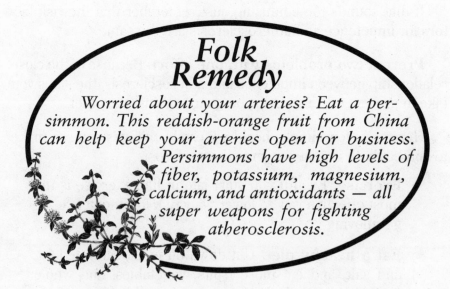

Folk Remedy

Worried about your arteries? Eat a persimmon. This reddish-orange fruit from China can help keep your arteries open for business. Persimmons have high levels of fiber, potassium, magnesium, calcium, and antioxidants — all super weapons for fighting atherosclerosis.

High blood pressure

Toss your blood pressure pills for good

Blood pressure drugs have undoubtedly prevented many deaths from heart disease and stroke in the last 30 years. According to a recent study, however, some people could do just as well without the drugs — if they're willing to make a few lifestyle changes.

Doctors sometimes prescribe medication to people with mild high blood pressure simply because they know most people won't follow their diet and exercise advice. If you only take one type of drug to treat mild high blood pressure, you may be able to stop buying those expensive little pills. Instead, you'll have to make lifestyle changes, such as maintaining an ideal body weight and following a low-salt, low-alcohol diet.

Of course, you should never stop taking any prescription drug without your doctor's approval. But if you would like to try lowering your blood pressure naturally, talk with him about these drug-free methods. Then, with his approval, try them.

What is it?

Blood pressure is the force of your blood pushing against your arteries. You suffer from high blood pressure when your heart must work harder than normal to pump blood through your circulatory system. This can damage both your heart and arteries and increase your risk of heart attack, stroke, kidney failure, eye damage, congestive heart failure, and atherosclerosis.

The top number of your blood pressure reading, your systolic pressure, is measured when your heart contracts. The bottom number, or diastolic pressure, is read when your heart relaxes.

Symptoms:

- No outer symptoms
- A blood pressure reading higher than 140/90

DASH it away. This eating plan came from a scientific study called Dietary Approaches to Stop Hypertension. The study compared three different eating plans, and the most effective plan became known as the DASH diet. It includes daily servings of four to five vegetables, four to five fruits, seven to eight grains, two to three low-fat or nonfat dairy products, two meats or less, and a half serving of nuts, seeds, or beans.

For more information about the DASH diet, visit the National Heart, Lung, and Blood Institute's Web site <www.nhlbi.nih.gov> or write to: NHLBI Health Information Center, P.O. Box 30105, Bethesda, MD 20824-0105.

Discover the Mediterranean way. Eat less fat, the experts say. But you can have your fat — within reason — and lower your blood pressure, too, if you eat like they do in Greece and southern Italy. A recent study found that people who replaced some of the saturated fat, like cream, butter, and cheese, in their diets with extra-virgin olive oil lowered their blood pressures significantly. Some were able to cut down on their blood pressure medicine or stop taking it altogether.

But according to the American Institute of Cancer Research, olive oil is only a small part of healthy eating in that part of the world. People in the Mediterranean eat a huge variety of plants — so much so that the people of Crete were once called "mangifolia," which means "leaf-eaters." Mediterranean people eat very little red meat or packaged foods, plenty of fish and vegetables, and drink a little red wine. Because variety is an important part of their diet, they eat small portions of many foods every day. The abundance of plant foods contributes lots of natural fiber, which has been linked to successful weight loss and good health. Who said a heart-healthy diet has to be boring?

Eat less, move more. Eating right is only half the battle when it comes to lowering blood pressure. Exercise provides the other half. A recent study found that a diet and exercise program not only lowered blood pressure, but also helped maintain that lower reading during times of mental stress. Losing as little as 3 percent of your body weight can help lower your blood pressure. If you weigh 200 pounds, you could have lower blood pressure after losing only six pounds. But why stop there? Keep going until you reach your ideal weight. Once your doctor clears you for exercise, get started right away. Try brisk walking if you haven't exercised in a while. As you tone up and slim down, you can ask your doctor about swimming, bicycling, and other forms of exercise.

Get the right mineral mix. While scientists disagree on whether a low-salt diet can lower blood pressure for everyone, you're probably getting a lot more of this mineral than you need. Try skimping on the salt for a while. If it turns out you're salt sensitive, your blood pressure should go down.

Other minerals, such as calcium, potassium, and magnesium, may help lower blood pressure. Low-fat dairy products offer you the best source of calcium. To get plenty of potassium, eat lots of fresh fruits, including avocados, bananas, figs, apricots, and cantaloupe. Beans, black-eyed peas, oysters, avocados, and sunflower seeds are good sources of magnesium.

Shake off bad habits. If you're worried about high blood pressure, you can make some lifestyle changes to decrease your risk. Don't smoke, and if you drink, limit your alcohol. That means no more than two drinks a day for a man, and one drink a day for a woman.

If you can manage to control your blood pressure without drugs, you'll save money and avoid unwanted side effects. Nevertheless, if you need to take medicine, don't hesitate. High blood pressure can have deadly results, and new research shows it even affects your thinking skills.

A sharp mind depends on a steady supply of oxygen-rich blood. Untreated high blood pressure can damage the inside of your arteries, hindering blood flow. To increase your powers of memory and concentration, keep your blood pressure under control.

Multi-talented mineral now easy to find

Thanks to the FDA's Halloween announcement, you'll find it easier to unmask foods masquerading as heart helpers.

On October 31, 2000, the FDA began allowing food manufacturers to make the following claim on certain products: "Diets containing foods that are good sources of potassium and low in sodium may reduce the risk of high blood pressure and stroke."

If you read that claim on food packaging, you can be sure the food in question contains the following:

- At least 10 percent of the recommended dietary allowance (RDA) of potassium, or 350 milligrams (mg)
- 140 mg or less of sodium
- Less than 3 grams of fat
- 1 gram or less of saturated fat
- 20 mg or less of cholesterol

The next time you're in the supermarket, keep your eyes open. You might find a great new food that's high in potassium and low in sodium, fat, and cholesterol — just the thing to give your high blood pressure a scare.

Shocking news about salt

For thousands of years, salt was a friend to man. People used it to keep meat, fish, and other foods from spoiling, and laborers ate it to replace minerals lost through sweat. But that was before refrigeration, air-conditioning, and cable TV.

Salt is a mineral composed of sodium and chloride. A sodium deficiency is harmful to your body, but very few diets are lacking in sodium. Your needs are small — about 500 milligrams (mg) a day, which is roughly one-quarter of a teaspoon of salt. The average person eats closer to 4,000 mg of sodium every day.

Maybe you've heard how salt can trigger high blood pressure in people who are salt sensitive. High blood pressure is a serious problem since it often leads to heart disease and increases your risk of an early death. New studies of salt and heart disease are even more worrisome. Scientists have found you can be salt sensitive without ever having high blood pressure. That means you are still at risk of dying from heart disease, but you won't have the warning sign of elevated blood pressure. And being overweight makes your risk even greater.

Because it's hard to test for salt sensitivity, the National Heart, Lung, and Blood Institute recommends everyone cut back to 2,400 mg of sodium a day, which is slightly more than one teaspoon of salt. That might sound like plenty, but salt adds up fast, especially in processed food.

"Only 10 percent of dietary sodium comes from salt added to food at the table," says Dr. Myron Weinberger, Director of the Hypertension Research Center at the Indiana University School of Medicine. "So to reduce their salt intake, Americans should be careful about the sodium content in prepared, preserved, and processed foods."

But food manufacturers know people like salt. That's why they've been slow to cut back, thinking you won't buy their food if it tastes a little different. Fast food is even worse. If your favorite fast-food meal is a Big Mac and large fries, that's a one-meal total of nearly 1,500 mg of sodium.

If you want to avoid heart disease, you'll have to check nutrition labels carefully for sodium content and change the way you eat. But with a little patience, you can actually enjoy a low-salt diet.

Be stingy. When you cook, try using half the salt called for in the recipe. It might be possible to cut salt completely from some recipes. You can always add a bit at the table. Just don't salt your food automatically, like many people do. At least taste food first, and

How much salt is hiding in your food?

Food	Sodium in milligrams
Meats:	
3 oz cooked roast beef	53
3 oz cooked chicken	50
1 large hot dog	638
3 oz chipped beef	2,953
Vegetables:	
1/2 cup cooked carrots	50
1 small baked potato	20
1 cooked ear of corn	3
1 cup creamed corn	572
Fruits:	
1 peach	0
1 cup canned peaches	16
1 slice peach pie	253
1 apple	0
1 slice apple pie	444
Fast and frozen food:	
TV dinner—chicken, corn, mashed potatoes, and chocolate pudding	1,820
Breakfast biscuit	1,470
Small cheeseburger	725
1 serving onion rings	800
Roast beef sandwich	792

if you feel it needs a little something, try pepper, onion or garlic powder, or a salt-free commercial product, like Mrs. Dash or Spike.

Make fresh choices. Buy fresh vegetables or look for low-sodium canned ones. After all these years, you might discover what green beans really taste like. Look for low-sodium soups, too, or make your own. Whenever possible, avoid processed meats, like cold cuts. And if something is labeled "pickled" or "cured," that means it's been soaked in salt, and you should avoid it. Even those oh-so-convenient rotisserie chickens in your grocery store are pre-treated with salt. To eat less salt, you'll have to do more cooking at home, but you'll be healthier for it.

Watch the extras. A lot of salt in your diet comes from condiments, like ketchup, mustard, steak and soy sauce, and extras like pickles. Would you believe a large dill pickle contains over 1,000 mg of salt? Munch on carrot sticks with your lunch, instead. Skip the high-sodium cup of soup with your sandwich, and try a side of vegetables or a salad. And don't even think about eating stuffing as a side dish anymore. One cup of stuffing is hiding over 1,000 mg of salt. Remember to check your drinks, too. A 12-ounce can of cola contains about 50 mg of sodium. Sip on water with a twist of lemon or lime.

Ask before you order. Eating out can be a challenge when you're on a special diet. Ask your waiter if the food you're ordering is prepared with salt or MSG, which is high in sodium. Many restaurants are able to cook your food the way you want it. Order sauces on the side and use them sparingly, or not at all, if they're salty.

Watch out for little-known hazards

You know that smoking, stress, and obesity can cause high blood pressure. But did you know a simple breakfast of coffee, toast, and orange marmalade could do the same thing?

173

In addition to the obvious high blood pressure risks, like fatty foods, alcohol, and salt, lurk other, lesser-known dangers. Here is just a small sampling of them, followed by some unusual methods of defense.

- ⬦ **Seville oranges.** These sour oranges, which crop up mostly in marmalade, have the same effect as grapefruit on your blood pressure medication. You've probably heard of the "grapefruit effect" or been warned not to take your medication with grapefruit or grapefruit juice. That's because grapefruit stops a certain enzyme from doing its job of metabolizing your medication. Without anything to stop it, the medication builds up in your body — possibly to toxic levels. Scientists recently discovered that the same thing happens with Seville oranges because, like grapefruit, they contain a substance called DHB. But since you're likely to eat Seville oranges only in marmalade — and a spoonful of marmalade probably doesn't contain enough DHB to affect your medication — the risk is small. Still, it might be a good idea not to take your blood pressure medication while you're munching on toast with orange marmalade.

- ⬦ **Coffee.** Some people can't imagine starting the day without a cup of java. Others enjoy just an occasional cup. Oddly, the part-timers might be at greater risk. Swiss doctors found that drinking coffee — even decaf — caused a big rise in blood pressure for people who usually don't drink coffee. While coffee stimulated the sympathetic nervous system in both groups, the usual coffee drinkers' blood pressure did not rise. Here's another coffee caution — stay away from it in times of stress if you have high blood pressure or a family history of the condition. A University of Oklahoma study showed that the combination of stress and caffeine sent blood pressure skyrocketing for these people, even if they were long-time coffee drinkers. In some cases, the blood pressure stayed high 12 hours after a single dose of caffeine.

↪ **Air pollution.** Smog alert! If you live in a big city, you're probably used to warnings when the air is particularly polluted. But now you might have another reason to be concerned about your environment. Turns out as air pollution gets worse, your blood pressure gets higher. German researchers discovered this trend, which hasn't been entirely explained. Pollutants in the air might affect the part of your nervous system that controls blood pressure. Air pollution also affects temperature, barometric pressure, and humidity — all factors that influence blood pressure. No matter what the reason, the problem is more serious for those who

Defeat dizziness with coffee

While coffee presents risks for people with high blood pressure, it can be a big help in certain short-term situations.

Here's an example. You eat dinner, then stand up from the table and feel lightheaded or dizzy.

It's a fairly common occurrence because your blood pressure drops after meals. This low blood pressure, or hypotension, may even cause you to faint.

Luckily, there's a simple solution. Drink a cup of coffee or tea right after your meal, and the caffeine will boost your blood pressure just enough to prevent these potentially dangerous symptoms.

Exercising does the same thing, and a post-meal stroll is a good way for younger people to ward off a temporary drop in blood pressure. But if you're older, your best bet is to drink a caffeinated beverage first. Once you feel stable on your feet, then go for a walk.

already have risk factors for heart disease, such as an increased heart rate. Their systolic blood pressure (the first number in a blood pressure reading) rose nearly four times more than that of other people. Heed those smog alerts, and limit your trips outside on especially bad days.

↜ **Licorice.** Chew on this disturbing news — snacking on licorice is no treat for your heart. A certain ingredient in licorice called glycyrrhizic acid wreaks havoc with your blood pressure. Researchers in Iceland found that eating as little as 50 grams of licorice, about the equivalent of a few jellybeans a day, could significantly raise your blood pressure. The good news is that most of the licorice sold in the United States is made with artificial flavoring, usually anise. But if real licorice is your favorite treat, you should probably cut down. And be on the lookout for real licorice in unexpected places, such as tobacco products and laxatives.

↜ **Cyclosporine.** This prescription drug, given to organ transplant recipients as well as people with rheumatoid arthritis and severe psoriasis, can cause high blood pressure. If your blood pressure shoots up while taking cyclosporine, your doctor will probably cut the dose by 25 to 50 percent. If the problem doesn't go away, you might have to switch medications.

↜ **Corticosteroids.** These steroids, which are similar to the natural hormone cortisone, can be used for a wide range of conditions, including skin problems, severe allergies, asthma, arthritis, eye diseases, organ transplants, and cancer. Unfortunately, these powerful anti-inflammatory drugs also cause you to retain salt and lose potassium, which can raise blood pressure. Over the short term and in small doses, corticosteroids rarely trigger any bad effects. But as your dosage and length of treatment increase, so does your risk of side effects. While taking corticosteroids, try to limit your salt intake and get more potassium into your diet. Good sources include dried apricots, avocados, figs, bananas, milk, and fish. Also, ask your doctor about alternate-day therapy where you only take your medication — at double the dose — every other morning. This sometimes cuts down on side effects. In any case, work with your doctor to make sure you're taking the lowest possible dose that still helps your condition.

Just as these unknown dangers can shift your blood pressure into overdrive, the following unorthodox methods can put the brakes on high blood pressure.

Mellow out with music. The next time you need minor surgery, such as for cataracts, play some tunes. A recent study found that music helped older people relax before and during surgery. Often, before undergoing surgery, your blood pressure builds to a crescendo because you're nervous. But when people in the study listened to music, their blood pressure levels went back to normal. It didn't even matter which type of music — symphony, big band, or even rock and roll. As long as they got to pick the music themselves, it seemed to work. The music made them feel more in control of the situation and helped distract them from what was happening. And if music can help lower blood pressure in a surgical setting, why not during other stressful times? Try music the next time you feel stressed. It might put your life, and your blood pressure, back in harmony.

Spend time with someone special. You'd never guess it from watching "The Honeymooners," but being around your spouse has a calming effect on your blood pressure. A study by Dr. Brooks B. Gump of the State University of New York at Oswego demonstrated that spending time with your spouse or a close friend helped lower blood pressure. It doesn't even matter what you're doing — just being around them makes a difference. It's probably because you feel safe and comfortable around people who are close to you. Oddly enough, even study participants who weren't satisfied with their partners had lower blood pressure when they spent time with them — although they didn't spend as much time with them. So no matter how busy your schedule might be, make some extra time for that special someone. After all, what's better for the heart than romance?

Outsmart mysterious silent killer

Many people feel anxious while being poked, prodded, and tested by someone in a white lab coat. That nervous tension often produces falsely high blood pressure readings dubbed "white-coat hypertension." But what about someone who is getting falsely low blood pressure readings in the doctor's office?

A recent study of 319 people revealed that 23 percent had this kind of high blood pressure. Called "white-coat normotension," it can only be detected during full-day monitoring. Older men who drink alcohol and are former smokers are at highest risk for this mysterious condition.

Here's how to make sure you don't have this hidden type of high blood pressure.

Check your numbers. Blood pressure readings between 130/80 and 150/100 are those most likely to be inaccurate. If you're in this questionable range, ask your doctor to take multiple readings. For better accuracy, request an ankle-arm ratio. This means measuring your blood pressure around your ankle as well as your upper arm. Your ankle-arm ratio — or the ankle reading divided by the arm reading — should be higher than 0.9. If it's not, it can mean serious heart trouble for you.

Take your own. To find out your real blood pressure, you'll need several readings taken throughout a normal day. You can take your own readings with the right equipment and training. But if your arm is bigger or smaller than average, don't even bother with the machines set up at drugstores. A study found that these machines did not accurately measure blood pressure in large or slim arms. Instead, they gave falsely high or low results.

To get a more precise reading, you can buy an electronic home blood pressure monitor, sold at most drugstores, and record your blood pressure every few hours. Follow the directions carefully and be sure the cuff fits properly. Before using the device, take it to your doctor, nurse, or pharmacist to make sure it works properly and you know how to use it.

Bone up on blood pressure. There are a few other things you should know about blood pressure and getting accurate readings.

- ✎ Make sure your cuff fits. A poorly fitting cuff can give a false reading — too high if it's very tight and too low if it's loose.

- ✎ Don't exert yourself before using the machine. This too will produce falsely high readings.

- ✎ Don't slump in your chair or talk while taking your blood pressure. Both can make your blood pressure rise.

- ✎ Sit comfortably and support your arm at about the level of your heart. An unsupported arm can give a higher reading.

- ✎ Blood pressure tends to be higher first thing in the morning and lower late at night. Blood pressure that doesn't drop in the late evening could be a symptom of other medical problems. Let your doctor know if you notice this pattern.

↦ If your blood pressure levels are consistently high, your doctor might want you to wear a small, electronic device that checks your blood pressure throughout the day. These automatic units do a thorough job of checking for high blood pressure. You'll also be scheduled for a follow-up visit to read and go over the results.

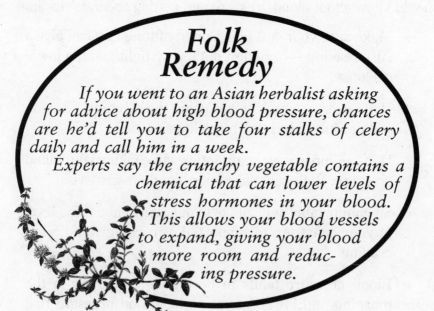

Folk Remedy

If you went to an Asian herbalist asking for advice about high blood pressure, chances are he'd tell you to take four stalks of celery daily and call him in a week.

Experts say the crunchy vegetable contains a chemical that can lower levels of stress hormones in your blood. This allows your blood vessels to expand, giving your blood more room and reducing pressure.

High cholesterol

Make 'heart smart' decisions about fats

Your doctor says your diet is your first line of defense against high cholesterol and heart disease. But how do you decide what to eat — especially when it comes to fats? Is butter better than margarine? Should you eat chocolate for the antioxidants or avoid it because of the high saturated fat content? How do you compare low-fat diets to high-protein diets, which may also be higher in fat?

Recent surveys show a lot of people, sad to say, are throwing up their hands in confusion and no longer worrying about fats. But your cholesterol level is far too important to ignore — so crucial, in fact, the government recently updated the guidelines for lowering it. One of the most important recommendations is to cut your daily saturated fat intake from 10 percent to 7 percent. If you're on a 1,500-calorie diet, that means you can have no more than 12 grams of saturated fat compared to 17 grams under the old rules. In food terms, that's about two-and-a-half homemade chocolate chip cookies.

But take heart. Choosing fats and adjusting your diet may not be as difficult as you think. You just

What is it?

Your body needs cholesterol to build cell walls, make hormones, and perform other important jobs, but too much of it can be dangerous. Since it can't dissolve in your blood, special particles called lipoproteins move this soft, waxy substance from place to place. Low-density lipoprotein (LDL) is the main cholesterol carrier. If you have too much LDL, over time cholesterol can build up on your artery walls (a condition called atherosclerosis), causing blockages and leading to heart attack or stroke. High-density lipoprotein (HDL) is known as "good" cholesterol because it carries cholesterol away from your arteries to your liver, where it is eliminated.

Symptoms:
- No outer symptoms
- Total cholesterol level over 200 mg/dl; LDL level over 130 mg/dl

need to understand that the kind of fat you eat may be as important as how much you eat.

Beware your heart's greatest enemy. That's saturated fat, found mainly in meats and full-fat dairy products like butter, cheese, and whole milk. It's the most dangerous fat because it raises your blood cholesterol and triglyceride levels, which increases your chances of clotting.

Saturated fat harms your arteries in a number of ways, warns Dr. Paul Nestel. Eating too much fat over time will build up damaging plaque in your blood vessels. And saturated fat wastes no time in making your arteries stiff and inflexible, say Nestel and fellow researchers at the Baker Medical Research Institute in Melbourne, Australia. Their study shows that eating a high-fat meal — 50 grams total, two-thirds from saturated fat — makes your arteries up to 27 percent less elastic within six hours. If your arteries can't stretch when blood pumps through them, it places a burden on your heart.

It's worth noting that the meal used in the study — a ham and cheese sandwich, a glass of whole milk, and ice cream for dessert — contained less fat than a typical meal of a cheeseburger and fries from a fast-food restaurant. So think twice before you ask for the super size at the drive-through window.

On the other hand, foods that contain saturated fat aren't all bad. Meat and cheese, for example, provide protein your body needs, and the antioxidants in chocolate may actually help your heart. Just be sure you don't go over the recommended 7 percent of your calories, and the benefits should outweigh the risks.

Go soft for a healthier diet. Polyunsaturated fats — like corn, safflower, sunflower, and sesame oils — stay liquid at room temperature and are better for you than saturated fats. The good news is they reduce your total cholesterol. Unfortunately, the good HDL drops right along with the bad LDL, and overuse may increase your risk of cancer.

Be especially leery of trans fatty acids found in hydrogenated vegetable shortenings and margarines. Although they are made from polyunsaturated fats, they undergo a process that makes them even worse for your arteries than saturated fats. They raise the LDL cholesterol and lower the HDL, which is doubly bad for your heart.

The harder these fats are at room temperature, the worse they are for your arteries. So stick to soft or liquid margarine, and eat fewer commercial baked goods, which are often made with hydrogenated fats.

Choose monounsaturated for more variety. If you find your low-fat diet getting monotonous, don't be discouraged. Dr. Penny Kris-Etherton believes using the right kind of fat will give you a variety of healthy diet choices. Monounsaturated fat — found in olive, canola, and peanut oils and in nuts — lowers your LDL cholesterol, but, unlike the polyunsaturated fats, does not lower your HDL. The new guidelines say your daily diet can contain 35 percent total fat — up from 30 percent — as long as it's mainly monounsaturated.

Kris-Etherton led a study at Penn State University that compared three diets high in monounsaturated fat to a low-fat diet and a typical American diet. The diets contained either 25-percent or 35-percent fat with almost half the fat in the "American" diet being saturated.

People in the study ate each of the diets for three and a half weeks. At the end of each period, researchers tested their blood to measure how fast the LDL oxidized — a signal that plaque was likely to build up in the arteries. The high-saturated-fat diet caused the fastest oxidation, while the rest oxidized LDL much more slowly.

"A Mediterranean style diet that focuses on fruit, vegetables, monounsaturated oil, nuts, legumes, and grain, and includes only small portions of meat would produce the beneficial changes seen in our study," Kris-Etherton says.

She also suggests other adjustments for a heart-healthy diet. "People could switch to low-fat dairy products," she notes. "Eat peanut butter instead of butter or full-fat cream cheese, use olive oil-based salad dressings, sprinkle nuts on vegetables instead of butter or margarine, and use nuts in salads or stews instead of meat." For those who really love the taste of beef, pork, or chicken in stews, she suggests substituting peanuts or other nuts for just part of the meat.

If you are still confused about fats, the chart on the next page should make it a little clearer.

Beat bad cholesterol with good nutrition

Need another reason to keep piling spinach and carrots on your dinner plate? Try lutein, a pigment found in green and yellow vegetables. Studies have already proven this nutrient is important for your eyes. Now research at the University of Southern California in Los Angeles shows it's good for your heart as well.

The study followed 480 middle-aged men and women for 18 months. During that time, those who had the most lutein in their bloodstream had almost no increase in the thickness of their carotid (neck) arteries. This was a good sign that the bad LDL cholesterol had not oxidized inside them and formed the dangerous plaque that can lead to heart attacks. Results of two other parts of the study, one done in the lab with human tissue and the other with mice, supported the findings of the first.

Dr. James Dwyer, who led this research, recommends eating plenty of lutein-rich foods to keep your arteries clear. "A diet rich in vegetables, including the dark green leafy variety," he says, "will provide sufficient lutein to achieve the levels of persons in our study."

Dwyer recommends at least one serving per day of foods like spinach, kale, collard greens, turnip greens, romaine lettuce, broccoli, zucchini squash, corn, brussels sprouts, and peas. But

Fats at a glance

Kind of Fat	Sources	Effect on cholesterol levels	Action advice
Saturated (solid at room temperature)	Meats, butter, lard, whole milk, cheese, palm kernel oil, coconut oil, chocolate	Raises both LDL and HDL cholesterol.	Limit to no more than 7 percent of calories daily. Eat lean cuts of meat and use low-fat dairy products.
Polyunsaturated (liquid at room temperature)	Vegetable oils: corn, safflower, sunflower, sesame, soybean, cottonseed	Reduces both HDL and LDL cholesterol. Too much may increase cancer risk.	Use oils and soft margarine in moderation, keeping total fat at or below 35 percent of calories per day.
Monounsaturated (liquid at room temperature)	Olive oil, peanut oil, canola oil, nuts, avocado	Lowers LDL. HDL stays the same or may be raised in some cases.	Use freely up to 35 percent of total calories per day.
Trans fatty acids (solid at room temperature)	Margarines, vegetable shortenings	Raises LDL. Lowers HDL.	Reduce or avoid commercially baked products (breads, cookies, cakes) and fried foods from fast-food restaurants. Look for recipes that offer other options in cooking.

he suggests you bypass the lutein supplements. The benefits of nutrients found in supplements, he points out, aren't always the same as those you get in foods and can even be risky.

"For example," he says, "vegetables rich in beta carotene are probably protective against some cancers, but beta-carotene supplements are toxic and increase the risk of lung cancer." Since the risks of lutein supplements haven't been determined yet, he suggests you stick to the vegetables.

Some doctors may advise those with kidney problems to avoid large quantities of leafy dark greens, Dwyer notes. But he doesn't think the research supports the fear these vegetables might increase kidney stones.

Lutein is just one way to use your diet to protect your heart. Here are some additional nutrients that will help keep your cholesterol in check, and aid in your fight against a number of other diseases as well.

Fiber. When it comes to lowering cholesterol and protecting your heart, saturated fat is the enemy and fiber is a hero. Fiber slashes LDL cholesterol while leaving the good HDL cholesterol alone. One six-year study involving more than 40,000 men found that, for every additional 10 grams of cereal fiber the men ate, their risk of heart disease decreased by an astounding 29 percent.

High-fiber foods are also more filling, which can help you lose weight and lower your risk of heart disease even more. To get lots of fiber, eat whole grains and fresh fruits and vegetables.

Magnesium. According to experts, most people get less than half the magnesium they need daily, and the consequences can be dangerous. Studies have linked magnesium deficiency to increased cancer risk, especially esophageal cancer.

Adding this mineral to your diet could lower your cholesterol by as much as one-third. And one study found that giving magnesium to people immediately after a severe heart attack cut their death rate in half during the critical four weeks following the attacks, when compared to heart attack victims who did not receive magnesium.

The recommended dietary allowance (RDA) for magnesium is 420 mg for men over 30 and 320 mg for women over 30. To reach this level, eat at least five servings of fresh or minimally processed fruits and vegetables daily. Avocados, sunflower seeds, pinto beans, spinach, oysters, and broccoli are especially good sources of this mineral.

Vitamin E. This fat-soluble vitamin may not lower cholesterol levels, but, like lutein, it can prevent LDL cholesterol from becoming oxidized and sticking to your artery walls. In one study, men who took at least 100 international units (IU) of vitamin E daily for at least two years had 37 percent fewer heart attacks than men who didn't take supplements. And a separate study found that women who took vitamin E supplements had 41 percent fewer heart attacks.

The RDA for vitamin E is 22 IU or 15 milligrams (mg). However, most studies that show a benefit to taking supplements used doses between 100 and 400 IU daily. Be sure to check with your doctor before taking more than the RDA of vitamin E, especially if you're taking blood-thinning medication. Good food sources of vitamin E include wheat germ oil, sunflower seeds, peanuts, mangoes, sweet potatoes, and olive oil.

Vitamin C. This is another antioxidant vitamin that helps prevent LDL cholesterol from becoming oxidized, and studies find it also helps raise HDL cholesterol levels.

Unlike vitamin E, however, vitamin C is a water-soluble vitamin, which means it isn't stored by your body. That makes it even more important to get as much of it as you need on a daily basis. Fortunately, that isn't difficult. Just one cup of orange juice gives you more than the RDA. Other good sources include sweet red peppers, green peppers, cantaloupe, brussels sprouts, grapefruit, and tomato juice.

Niacin. This B vitamin works so well to lower cholesterol, doctors prescribe it as a treatment. However, high doses can cause itching, flushing, rash, and stomach pain as well as more serious side effects such as ulcers, liver damage, and symptoms of diabetes. To get your niacin naturally, eat tuna, chicken, liver, salmon, potatoes, and beans.

Head off heart attacks from hidden fat

Watch out for a little-known danger that may sneak up on you while you are busy focusing on your cholesterol. Triglycerides, an equally dangerous fat, may be just waiting to strike. One study found your risk of having a heart attack is three times greater if you have high triglycerides compared to those with normal levels.

Triglycerides are fats that provide most of the fuel for your body. You get some from the fat in your diet, and your liver makes the rest from the carbohydrates you eat. Like all fats, they are necessary, within limits, for good health. But studies have found a link between elevated triglyceride levels and heart disease. And high triglycerides and high LDL cholesterol together deal a double whammy to your heart's health.

On the other hand, the combination of low triglycerides and high HDL cholesterol is a plus. It puts you at less risk for heart disease even if your LDL cholesterol is high. Unfortunately, a good HDL level alone won't protect you if your triglycerides are out of sight. And if triglyceride problems run in your family, you're more likely to die from a heart attack even when your blood cholesterol is normal, says Melissa A. Austin, Ph.D., a researcher at the University of Washington. She and her colleagues looked at the medical histories of more than 100 families over 20 years and found that high triglyceride levels could predict heart attacks years in advance.

Fortunately, a few lifestyle changes may be all you need to get your triglycerides under control. Similar to those for lowering

Save your heart with substitutes

Chicken eggs are good sources of protein, vitamin E, and unsaturated fatty acids, but they also contain about 200 mg of cholesterol each. If you're worried about heart disease, it makes sense to limit the number you eat. But don't forget to count the eggs in baked goods. Try the following egg substitutes when baking to keep your cholesterol levels down.

- For each egg called for, mix together 1 1/2 tablespoons of water, 1 1/2 tablespoons of oil, and 1 teaspoon of baking powder.
- Stir 1 envelope of unflavored gelatin into 1 cup of boiling water. Store in your refrigerator, and microwave the mixture when you want to use it. For each egg, substitute 3 tablespoons of the liquid.

cholesterol, these strategies will help slash your troublesome triglycerides and keep your risk for heart disease low.

Maintain a healthy weight. One of the most important things you can do for your heart is to keep your weight in a healthy range by balancing the calories you take in with those you burn. Your body converts extra calories to triglycerides and stores them, increasing your chances of heart disease.

Increase physical activity. Regular exercise can help you reach that ideal balance of high HDL and low triglycerides.

Limit sugar and white breads. Eat more whole grains and keep sweets to a minimum in your diet. Refined carbohydrates — like baked goods made with white flour — and simple carbohydrates — like sugar, honey, corn syrup, and molasses — can raise your triglycerides.

Reduce saturated fat in your diet. Avoid fatty cuts of meats and full-fat dairy products. But don't cut your total fat to less than

15 percent of your daily calories. According to the American Heart Association, going lower can increase your triglycerides and reduce your HDL cholesterol, just the opposite of what you want.

The latest government guidelines on cholesterol recommend keeping your fat intake under 35 percent of your daily calories. Replace saturated fats with healthier ones — like the monounsaturated fats found in olive, canola, and peanut oils, as well as avocados and nuts.

Know your heart disease risk

Changes in the cholesterol guidelines mean you may now be in a category that requires treatment, either through diet or drugs. To understand your risk for heart disease, you need to know more than just your total cholesterol level. The experts at the National Institutes of Health (NIH) recommend you get a full lipoprotein analysis — which includes your LDL, HDL, and triglyceride levels — every five years.

Here are the numbers you should aim for:
- Total cholesterol: Below 200 mg/dL
- LDL cholesterol: Below 100 mg/dL
- HDL cholesterol: Above 60 mg/dL
- Triglycerides: Below 150 mg/dL

If your cholesterol levels are borderline, you may be able to lower them through lifestyle changes rather than drugs. Besides eating less saturated fat and cholesterol, you should lose weight if needed, exercise, eat more fiber, and use cholesterol-lowering spreads instead of butter. Talk to your doctor about the right treatment for you.

For a copy of the full NIH cholesterol report, go to the Web site <www.nhlbi.nih.gov/guidelines/cholesterol/index.htm>. Or send a request for NIH Publication No. 01-3670 to the U.S. Department of Health and Human Services, National Institutes of Health, Bethesda MD 20892.

Feed on fiber. Eating whole grains, dried beans and other fibrous vegetables, and fruits with their skins will help lower triglycerides. But don't count on the same good results from fiber supplements.

Eat more fatty fish. Salmon, albacore or blue fin tuna, sardines, lake trout, and mackerel are healthy sources of omega-3 fatty acids. These, and fish oil supplements as well, can help lower triglycerides.

Don't smoke. The fact that it appears to raise triglycerides is just one of many reasons not to smoke.

Watch your alcohol intake. Although moderate drinking seems to benefit your heart in some ways, it can also increase your triglycerides if they are already high. If you drink, stay at or below the recommended daily limit of two drinks — containing one-half ounce of pure alcohol — if you are a male and one drink if you are a female.

If you find these lifestyle changes don't lower your triglycerides to 150 or below — considered normal under the new government guidelines — talk to your doctor about medications that can help. Besides putting you at risk for heart disease, high triglycerides could be a sign of diabetes, an under-active thyroid, kidney disease, or some other serious health problem.

Spread the good news about fake fats

You may love buttered toast for breakfast, but you know it's not exactly a heart-healthy way to start your day. Of course, choosing whole-grain bread will give you a good dose of cholesterol-lowering fiber, but butter is high in saturated fat, and a pat of trans-fatty margarine may be even worse.

Fortunately, your supermarket dairy case holds a couple of healthy alternatives, according to the National Institutes of Health (NIH). Instead of butter or margarine, choose Benecol Spread, a fat

Search family tree for cholesterol clues

If you eat low-fat foods and follow other recommendations to keep cholesterol low, but your LDL level is still high, you may have familial hypercholesterolemia. Untreated, this inherited condition can dramatically increase your risk of heart disease. Fortunately, your doctor can prescribe effective medications, but the earlier you start treatment the better.

Researcher Dr. Andrew Neil of the University of Oxford in England points out that this kind of high cholesterol frequently is not diagnosed until later in life. Unfortunately, his research shows about half of the men and a third of the women who have it will suffer a heart attack by age 60 if they don't get it under control.

And it's important not to stop with your own treatment. "If a patient is diagnosed as having familial hypercholesterolemia," says Neil, "it is essential that their first degree relatives be screened to determine whether they are affected."

So if you have this condition, tell your parents, brothers and sisters, and children about it so they can be tested, too. Treatment with diet and drugs, if needed, can begin even in childhood to lower the risk of serious heart problems.

substitute recently endorsed by the Food and Drug Administration (FDA) for its cholesterol-lowering ability. Or try Take Control, another spread that gives you the same heart-healthy benefits.

New NIH guidelines for lowering cholesterol recommend 2 grams of plant stanols, found in Benecol; or sterols, found in Take Control, every day. Both substances work by blocking your body's absorption of cholesterol. Read the label to see how much of the spread you'll need to get the suggested amount.

Other fat substitutes allow you to enjoy an occasional high-fat snack without worrying that your cholesterol level will skyrocket.

Olestra, for example, takes potato chips off the high-danger list. It can't increase your cholesterol because your body won't digest it, but it may cause some unpleasant side effects in your intestinal tract. And chips, no matter what they're made of, aren't particularly healthy, so think twice before using them to replace nutritious snacks like fruit.

Hydrogenated oils, used by the ton in fast-food restaurants, are guaranteed to harden your arteries. Once again, a product has come to the rescue that makes fried foods a little safer to eat. Appetize is a blend of corn oil and beef tallow with the natural cholesterol removed. Research suggests it also may help lower blood cholesterol.

Unfortunately, fast-food restaurants aren't rushing to replace their artery-clogging fats with this substitute. Until they do, go easy on the burgers and fries, and try to eat more meals at home where you can take advantage of healthy fat substitutes.

Folk Remedy

Europeans have used artichokes for centuries for all sorts of illnesses, including those of the heart and blood. Scientists now know that an ingredient in artichokes, called cynarin, helps lower cholesterol. In fact, cynarin extract is currently used in cholesterol-lowering drugs.

Why not go straight to the source for a tasty treat that can lower high cholesterol? Add artichokes to your plate a few times each week. Just watch what you dip the leaves in. A rich, buttery sauce will do your cholesterol more harm than good. Try a yogurt-based dip instead.

Stroke

Lifestyle strategies help sidestep strokes

It's Monday morning and many people have another reason to feel blue — more strokes happen on Mondays than on any other day. Some of the blame goes to those weekend activities, which might include a physical workout, or heavier than usual smoking and drinking. In addition, Monday morning often means going back to a stressful job.

Since you can't tear Mondays off your calendar, check out these lifestyle choices that can influence your stroke risk.

Say no more butts. If you smoke, quit. It's the most important change you can make to protect yourself from heart disease. Out of alcohol use, smoking, weight, and diet, smoking had the greatest influence on the risk of serious health problems, including heart disease and strokes. Ask your doctor to recommend a program to help you stop smoking. Try a nicotine patch or special gum — anything to kick the habit. Just don't wait another day.

Bank some blood. One of the blessings of living in a prosperous country is having plenty to eat. Unfortunately, it's also one of the curses. Because you have access to unlimited amounts of meat and other sources of protein, chances are you have too much iron stockpiled in your blood. People with higher stores of iron tend to get worse after having a stroke, and they suffer more brain damage than other stroke victims.

If you're in good health, stop by the next blood drive in your town. By donating blood, you'll reduce the amount of iron in your body and do a good deed in the process.

Change that spare tire. Extra weight makes your heart work harder, makes you more vulnerable to heart disease, and increases your risk of stroke. For every six or seven pounds you gain, your stroke risk rises by 6 percent. Ask yourself if that large serving of fries or that piece of chocolate cake is really worth it. Stick to a sensible, low-fat diet high in fruits, vegetables, and whole grains, and you'll see those extra pounds — and your risk of stroke — melt away.

Move those muscles. Do your arteries need a good workout? If you have heart disease they certainly do. Just by pedaling an exercise bicycle for 10 minutes, six times a day, men with narrowed or hardened arteries increased the amount of blood that flowed to their hearts.

Exercise helps the cells that line your blood vessels expand, allowing better and faster circulation.

Opt for optimism. Keep on the sunny side of life, the old song says. Have this as your philosophy, and you're likely to live longer and experience fewer health problems. According to researchers at the University of Texas Medical Branch at Galveston, happy people are less likely to have strokes.

If cheerfulness comes easily to you, congratulations. However, if you often feel sad or depressed, you might have a chemical imbalance. This kind of physical problem can be corrected. Visit your doctor for tests.

> ## *What is it?*
>
> A stroke, sometimes called a "brain attack," can damage your brain the way a heart attack harms your heart. Some are caused by blood clots that block the flow of blood to the brain (an ischemic stroke). Others happen when a blood vessel in the brain ruptures (a hemorrhagic stroke). When the cells in your brain are deprived of oxygen in your blood, they die — and never come back. As with a heart attack, fast action can save your life.
>
> Symptoms:
> - Numbness or weakness, especially on one side
> - Confusion, trouble speaking or understanding
> - Difficulty seeing
> - Dizziness, loss of balance or coordination
> - A sudden, severe headache

You can also see a trained counselor or psychologist for further insight into your mood. Sometimes just talking about your problems can lighten the load and your outlook. For your heart's sake, exercise your constitutional right and pursue happiness.

Stop stroke hook, line, and sinker

A fish a day could make stroke go away — almost.

Let's say you eat fish at least five times a week. You've just cut your risk of suffering a stroke in half. That's a whale of a finding.

Stroke symptoms = the need for speed

If you or someone you love suddenly can't talk or think clearly, or has a blinding headache, weakness, or paralysis, call for emergency help. Don't waste precious time searching for an available relative or friend to drive you to the hospital. Emergency medical technicians know to act quickly and efficiently, and they won't panic as a neighbor or relative might. You have a better chance of survival if you get help at the first sign of stroke symptoms.

In addition, a new medicine, called tPA, works to dissolve the clots causing an ischemic stroke. It can dramatically increase your odds of making a full recovery, but it will only help if it's given within three hours of the first symptoms.

"Currently, only about 5 percent of stroke patients arrive at the hospital in time to receive tPA because most people don't know the warning signs or don't realize they should seek medical help immediately," says Edgar J. Kenton, III, M.D., chair of the American Stroke Association Advisory Committee.

If the unthinkable does happen, don't panic — act quickly and get to the hospital fast. Doctors need that time to order tests and prescribe the proper treatment.

These promising numbers come out of a recent study published in the *Journal of the American Medical Association*. During the course of 14 years, researchers from the Harvard Medical School and the University of Miami School of Medicine followed the eating habits of almost 80,000 women. They came to the conclusion the more fish they ate, the better chance they had of living stroke-free.

Men can net the same benefits. If you eat about an ounce or more of fish per day, you'll have half the risk of stroke as men who reel in less fish. It takes just two delicious filets a week to meet this quota.

The heroes behind these true-to-life fish tales are compounds you probably have heard about before — omega-3 fatty acids that keep blood clots from forming. With names like eicosapentaenoic acid (EPA) and docosahexaenoic acid (DHA), it's easier to eat omega-3 fatty acids than spell them. The best way to do that is by choosing cold-water, fatty fish like anchovies, bluefish, herring, mackerel, mullet, salmon, sardines, sturgeon, trout, tuna, and whitefish.

Actually, some experts believe fish oil is such a powerful anti-clot compound that too much could be dangerous, increasing your risk of hemorrhagic stroke — when blood vessels in your brain rupture and cause internal bleeding.

You don't really have to worry about this, however. Eating like an Eskimo once in a while, according to the Harvard-Miami researchers, does not appear to put you at greater risk for hemorrhagic strokes. For real danger, you would have to eat fish at least three times every day — getting around 3 grams of omega-3 fatty acids.

If any amount of fish is too much for you, get omega-3 fatty acids from landlubber foods. Try flaxseed, walnuts, and dark leafy greens like collard, spinach, arugula, Swiss chard, and kale.

By including these foods in your regular diet, you'll not only protect your brain from stroke, but also guard against arthritis, skin problems, immune system imbalances, and depression.

Guard against food-drug interactions

Blood thinners could save your life — or end it. This type of medication protects many people from life-threatening blood clots. But certain foods and herbs interact with blood thinners like warfarin, putting you in danger of a particular type of life-threatening stroke.

If you have a family history of hemorrhagic stroke — when a blood vessel in your brain ruptures — and if you take warfarin, you must be especially careful to avoid these deadly interactions. In addition, if you have high blood pressure, you're more at risk of a hemorrhagic stroke since the walls of your blood vessels are weak and more likely to burst.

Learn what can interact with warfarin, and talk to your doctor about your risk.

Vitamin K. You need this vitamin for your blood to clot properly, but when paired with warfarin, it can spell trouble. A single large intake of vitamin K can block warfarin and cause dangerous blood clots. Don't cut out all foods rich in K — just don't go to extremes. Eat foods like broccoli, brussels sprouts, kale, parsley, spinach, egg yolks, liver, and vegetable oils on a regular schedule. For instance, eat three servings of broccoli each week — not six servings one week and none the next. Also, avoid taking large doses of vitamin K supplements without the approval of your doctor.

Garlic. The same compounds that make this spice a superstar heart healer could also make it dangerous for people taking blood thinners. Garlic naturally stops your blood from clotting. Taking two blood thinners at once — your medication and garlic — could lead to uncontrollable bleeding. That spells hemorrhagic stroke if it occurs in your brain. To avoid this, experts warn against taking standardized garlic extract. They also suggest eating no more than one clove of garlic a day.

Ginkgo. In a few isolated cases, mixing warfarin and ginkgo has led to dangerous internal bleeding. That's because ginkgo, like garlic, keeps your blood cells from clumping together and forming clots. So, before you take ginkgo, talk with a doctor or pharmacist.

Vitamin E. This vitamin, by itself, is a blood thinner. Combine it with warfarin and you run the risk of thinning your blood too much. Play it safe by avoiding large doses of vitamin E — over 400 International Units (IU) a day — while you're on warfarin. Eat E-rich foods like avocados, nuts, seeds, and wheat germ in moderation.

Papaya. A compound in papaya, called papain, could also make warfarin's effects stronger. So, ask your doctor before you eat papaya or take products with papain in them.

When the thrill can kill

Imagine that first drop on a roller coaster, the one so steep you can't even see where it ends. It's enough to scare some people to death — and for good reason. That brain-jarring plunge, and all the twists and turns that follow, can bring on a fatal stroke.

Most people handle roller coasters with little more than a queasy stomach. But in some cases, the speed and force of the ride can actually cause bleeding inside your brain, which could lead to a stroke.

You're especially at risk if you suffer from frequent headaches, atherosclerosis, high blood pressure, any other serious heart problem or brain disorder, or if you take blood-thinning medication like warfarin.

In these cases, your safest bet is to stay off the ride. However, if you just can't give up the thrill, beware of the main sign of trouble — a headache afterward. See your doctor immediately if one occurs.

Alcohol. Alcohol can cause your body to process blood thinners more rapidly. An occasional drink shouldn't be a problem, but don't dramatically change your drinking habits while you're on warfarin. And always drink in moderation.

Warfarin reacts with a wide variety of over-the-counter and prescription medications. Be careful with aspirin, acetaminophen, antibiotics, and certain drugs for high cholesterol and ulcers. Ask your doctor how much — if any — is safe to take.

Snap back from stroke

Millions of people survive strokes. It's a tough road back to your former life, but with determination — and help — you can walk that road.

After a stroke, you'll face physical and emotional obstacles. You may need to learn new ways to perform day-to-day activities. You must cope with fatigue and depression. But as serious as these side effects are, remember, you aren't helpless and you aren't alone.

Send your body back to school. Even if your stroke happened 20 to 30 years ago, an innovative new treatment called constraint-induced therapy (CIT) could bring strength and coordination back to crippled limbs. CIT involves forcing you to use your weakened arm, hand, or leg. Sometimes the "good" limb is restricted in some way — even tied down. Your brain relearns how to move and control the disabled limb.

According to Dr. Richard D. Zorowitz, Director of Stroke Rehabilitation with the University of Pennsylvania Health System, CIT is very effective, especially for stroke survivors with chronic problems.

"The key to CIT," he says, "is using the affected limb as much as possible."

For over 300 stroke sufferers, CIT has already given them close to their original strength. Talk to your doctor about how this therapy can help you become more independent.

Swallow with care. Losing your ability to swallow is a condition called dysphagia. It can lead to dehydration, malnutrition, and even pneumonia caused by inhaling food or liquid.

If you chew or swallow more slowly than before, or if eating feels like a workout, you could have dysphagia. Ask your doctor to recommend a speech or language pathologist. She'll give you specific exercises to improve strength and coordination in your face and neck.

Also, try these self-help tips.

- Eat sitting up or leaning forward with your chin either parallel to the table or tucked down.

- Start your meal with something icy and repeat any time you begin to have swallowing problems during a meal.

- Don't try to wash solid food down with a liquid.

- Choose soft, moist foods and thick liquids. Avoid dry foods and thin liquids.

- Swallow twice for each mouthful of solid food.

- Swallow, clear your throat, and swallow again for each mouthful of liquid.

- Hold your breath when you swallow anything.

- Stick with purées or easily chewed foods.

- Take only small sips and bites.

- Use liquid thickeners from your local pharmacy.

According to Zorowitz, up to one-third of stroke survivors suffer from dysphagia. Fortunately, many recover naturally — sometimes within the first month following a stroke.

Don't lose sleep over sneezes. Sometimes a stroke damages the "sneeze center" in your brain. As unbelievable as it sounds, you could become temporarily powerless to sneeze. While this reflex should return in time, avoid dusty places and tell your doctor.

Put on a happy face. Depression is a common result of stroke, however, feeling hopeless can keep you from recovering your life and your health. There are several reasons why you're glum.

"Chemical imbalances that can occur as a result of stoke cause the depression sometimes," Zorowitz says. For other stroke survivors, the stress and frustration of recovery can be too much to bear. And now, experts are suggesting that your personality before the stroke influences your emotional recovery. If you were moody and withdrawn before, you're likely to be less interested in rehabilitation. If you were outgoing and social, you're more likely to make a better recovery and get on with your life in an easier fashion.

Whatever your personality, get help if you feel depressed after a stroke. "Know you're not alone," Zorowitz says. Share your feelings with loved ones, your doctor, or a therapy group. Continue to take part in the hobbies and activities that bring you pleasure. And be proud of any progress you make, no matter how small.

Don't forget, depression after a stroke is usually temporary. As you recover and become more independent, you'll find happiness again.

Fight off fatigue. One of the toughest side effects of stroke is fatigue. Having low energy levels is a problem in itself, but it can also make depression and physical difficulties that much harder to handle. The first step to overcoming fatigue is talking about it with your doctor and loved ones.

Then, don't overwhelm yourself during times of the day when you're most tired. "Being in tune with your body makes a difference," Zorowitz says. Take care of important daily tasks when you feel up to it. Then, if you have energy left over, handle less important things. Above all, rest in between activities to recharge your batteries. "Build your endurance," says Zorowitz.

Balance your life. Continue leading the healthy lifestyle you had before your stroke. That means eat right and exercise. Both habits will help you cope with depression, stress, and fatigue. If eating is a problem, ask your doctor about supplements. If it's difficult to exercise, simply try to stay as independent as possible — that can be a workout in itself.

INSOMNIA

Sleep to prevent health nightmares

You've heard the expression "You snooze, you lose." Well, the opposite is actually true. You have much more to lose — your good health and possibly even your life — if you don't snooze.

Experts explain the danger with the term "sleep debt." Any time you don't get enough sleep — on average eight hours a night for adults — you accumulate sleep debt. For example, short-changing yourself of one hour's sleep each night for eight nights in a row adds up to a sleep debt of eight hours — the same effect as if you'd skipped an entire night's sleep. This kind of sleep deprivation can lead to all kinds of health problems.

Stay on the ball. Sleep-deprived drivers are just as dangerous as drunk drivers, if not more so. Lack of sleep dulls your intellect, motor skills, and reaction time, making you more likely to have an accident. One study showed people who had been awake for 17 to 19 hours (a normal day for some people) had reaction times 50 percent slower than those of people legally drunk. Sleep experts say if you need to catch up on some shuteye, keep your naps to about 20 minutes.

Fine-tune the time change. Daylight savings time poses a special risk because everyone has been cheated out of an hour's sleep. In fact, you're five times more likely to have an accident on the day after you "spring ahead." To remedy this danger, gradually adjust to the time change over the course of a week rather than all at once. In other words, ease — don't spring — ahead. Go to bed 10 minutes earlier and get up 10 minutes earlier each day in the week leading up to the time change. By then, your body will be adjusted, so you won't miss that "lost" hour.

Protect your personal life. Not getting enough sleep puts your body under added stress. Your memory suffers, and you might become testy or withdrawn from family and friends — not to mention too tired to enjoy leisure or social activities.

The problem extends to the bedrooms of married couples. Results of the National Sleep Foundation survey show more than half of Americans are having sex less often than they did five years ago. Of those with marital difficulties, about half are sleeping less and three-fourths have sleep problems.

Experts recommend using your bed only for sleeping and sex. In addition, make the bedroom comfortable — not too hot or too cold, with soft, restful lighting. Finally, establish regular bed and waking times.

Hang on to your health. Besides your driving, work performance, and personal relationships, sleep deprivation also takes its toll on your health. Dr. Eve Van Cauter of the University of Chicago measured insulin production in healthy, but sleep-deprived people.

What is it?

Insomnia, the inability to fall asleep and stay asleep, can lead to physical, mental, emotional, and safety problems. Worry is probably the most common cause, but sleep apnea, restless legs syndrome, or too much light or noise in your bedroom are sometimes to blame. Certain medications and lifestyle choices including too little exercise or drinking too much coffee can also keep you awake.

Symptoms:
- Daytime drowsiness
- Fatigue
- Irritability
- Difficulty coping

She found that those who slept about five hours per night produced 50 percent more insulin than those who slept about eight hours a night. They also showed 40 percent lower insulin sensitivity than the normal sleepers. Lower insulin sensitivity puts you at greater risk for diabetes. It can also lead to obesity and high blood pressure, risk factors for a wide range of problems, including heart disease and stroke.

If you cut out late-night snacking, exercise daily, and limit caffeine, alcohol, and smoking in the evening, you'll not only sleep better, but perhaps live longer, too.

Sleep debt is a growing problem. A recent survey conducted by the National Sleep Foundation reports that 63 percent of American adults get less than eight hours' sleep. People are working more and sleeping less, a dangerous combination for your health. Remember, the only way to pay back sleep debt is to sleep.

Let sunlight lull you to sleep

Contrary to popular belief, insomnia isn't a natural part of old age. True, as you get older your body may produce less melatonin — a hormone that helps you sleep — but you might be making the problem worse if you don't get enough sunlight.

A recent Japanese study compared nursing home residents with insomnia to residents without sleeping problems and to healthy college students. When researchers made sure the elderly insomniacs got an extra four hours of bright light a day, their nighttime melatonin levels increased to match those of the young group. Their sleeping patterns also improved.

When sunlight affects your melatonin levels, it also affects your body's internal clock — the mechanism that tells you when it's time to sleep and when it's time to wake up. So, before you turn to sleeping pills or other drugs, try these simple, natural sunlight remedies.

Get outdoors. What better way to get sunlight than by enjoying a pleasant day outside? Take a walk around the block. Not only will you help yourself by getting more sunlight, you'll also get some exercise. Often, too little exercise can cause insomnia.

Sit in a sunny room. If you prefer to spend your day indoors, sit in a room that lets in plenty of sunlight. You can read, solve a crossword puzzle, watch television, or do whatever activity you want. Just by moving to a room on the sunny side of the house, you might get the extra sunlight you need.

Open it up. Your current room might be sunny enough — if you just keep your curtains open and your window shades up. Privacy is important, but so is your sleep. Even if it's just for a couple hours a day, invite the sun into your home for a visit.

Rise and shine. In the Japanese study mentioned earlier, the elderly insomniacs were exposed to bright midday sun — from 10 a.m. to noon and from 2 p.m. to 4 p.m. However, some evidence suggests early morning sun is best for changing your body's internal clock. This strategy can help people with Seasonal Affective Disorder (SAD), a form of depression brought about by the change in seasons.

Keep in mind not all light is good for you. Experts say getting too much artificial light just before bed can disrupt your internal clock and lead to sleeping troubles.

Stifle snoring for better slumber

Snoring does more than just disrupt your spouse's sleep. It can also present health problems, especially if it means you have sleep apnea. This condition causes you to temporarily stop breathing during the night. You wake up often, sometimes gasping for air. With so much interrupted sleep, you often feel tired and rundown during the day.

Since sleep apnea is a potentially dangerous condition, visit your doctor for the proper diagnosis. Then, if you're looking for ways to enjoy a nice, quiet night of slumber, check out these remedies.

Shed your clothes for sounder sleep

Wearing undergarments to bed may not be such a good idea.

If you have a habit of keeping on your bra or girdle all night, you're probably robbing yourself of deep, restful sleep.

In a clinical study, wearing a bra and girdle for the final 24 hours of a three-night study, lowered melatonin levels and raised body temperatures. These two automatic functions not only influence each other, but also determine how well you sleep. Experts believe tight undergarments can cause body changes by putting pressure on your skin and constricting your blood vessels.

For the sweetest sleep, make sure your nightclothes are loose and comfortable.

Get a handle on hormones. Men are three times more likely to have sleep apnea than women. However, once women go through menopause, their rate of sleep apnea increases dramatically. Hormone replacement therapy (HRT) — especially containing both estrogen and progesterone — appears to lower that risk.

Experts aren't entirely sure why HRT works, but they suspect it has something to do with the link between snoring and hormones. There are general health controversies surrounding hormone replacement and it's definitely not for everyone. Before you make a decision, talk to your doctor and learn the pros and cons.

Grab a gadget. More than 300 anti-snoring products are patented with the U.S. Patent and Trademark Office. Just be careful of bogus products that sound too good to be true. Many of them are scams that will take your money but won't do a thing for your snoring problem. On the other hand, some anti-snoring devices actually work. Talk to your doctor about all your options.

You may want to try something called a continuous positive airway pressure mask. You wear it over your nose or mouth when you sleep. It blows air into your nasal passages, keeping the airways open.

Ask your dentist or orthodontist about fitting you for a special oral or dental appliance. These work best for mild to moderate sleep apnea.

The Federal Trade Commission (FTC) investigates misleading advertising claims and tries to protect the public from sham businesses and their products. If you have a question about an anti-snoring product, call the FTC at 1-877-FTC-HELP or visit their Internet site at <www.ftc.gov>.

Have a ball. One cheap and effective anti-snoring device is a simple tennis ball. Sew one or two to the back of your pajamas and you'll find it difficult to sleep on your back — the position that makes you most likely to snore. Sleeping on your back also leads to more frequent and severe sleep apnea events.

Pop in to the pharmacy. Enter a drugstore, and the number of over-the-counter anti-snoring products might overwhelm you. At least one homeopathic remedy did improve snoring in a clinical trial, but that doesn't mean every product works. Ask your doctor or pharmacist before trying any non-prescription treatment.

Change your lifestyle. No matter how many gizmos, gimmicks, and gadgets are out there, you'll deal with snoring best by changing your daily routine. Lose weight if you're overweight. Treat your high blood pressure. Avoid alcohol right before bedtime. Sleep on your side. These steps are simple, safe, and healthy. Give them a try — you might silence both your snoring and your spouse's complaints.

Keep surgery in mind. A legitimate option for serious sleep apnea, surgery can help by widening your airway. But, according to a recent study, it's often unnecessary and unhelpful.

People who undergo a laser procedure called uvulopalatoplasty, which removes excess tissue in your throat, often relapse and start snoring again after a few months. In some cases, surgery even makes the snoring worse. Experts say for best results, it's critical patients return for follow-up treatments.

Another procedure, radiofrequency tissue volume reduction (RFTVR), uses a needle electrode and radio frequencies to burn your soft palate tissue, causing it to shrink and stiffen. RFTVR is a fairly painless, simple treatment that's shown some success. It's still new, however, and hasn't been thoroughly tested.

Remember, surgery should be a last option. Explore other treatments first.

Wake up your tired eyes

If eyes are truly the windows to your soul, make sure they show the real you and not the remnants of a sleepless night.

Lack of sleep can make your eyes baggy, saggy, and puffy. And then there are those dark circles. Before you reach for the sunglasses, try these natural tips to make your eyes look and feel clear and rested.

Calm them with cucumber. One of the oldest beauty tricks in the book really works. Slap a slice of cold cucumber on each eye and relax for a few minutes.

Take a tea break. Say so long to puffy eyes with a couple of cold, wet tea bags. Tea contains tannins, an astringent that can tighten your skin, and caffeine, which will constrict the blood vessels. Anyone who's ever peeked in a teapot knows that tea can stain, so it may a good idea to wrap the teabag in tissue to keep it from discoloring your skin.

Crack open an egg. Plain old egg whites are a farm-fresh alternative to expensive facial masks. Just apply the whites to your face with a makeup brush. As the egg whites dry, your skin will tighten up, including that saggy area under your eyes.

Come around with a compress. When all else fails, a cold, wet washcloth will soothe your eyes and reduce swelling. If you're hardy enough, place the cloth in the freezer for a while to chill it thoroughly.

Be a potato head. Some say the potassium in raw potato slices can lighten the dark circles under your eyes.

Pile up the pillows. That puffiness sometimes comes from fluid collecting under your eyes while you sleep. Try using an extra pillow at night to elevate your head. And don't sleep on your stomach — you may get fewer wrinkles.

Shake the habit. If you're retaining fluid, you may get swollen eyes more often. Go easy on the saltshaker and limit caffeine and alcohol, especially right before bedtime.

For good general skin care, get plenty of rest. If your eyes are often swollen, red, or itchy, you may have allergies or another medical condition. See your doctor.

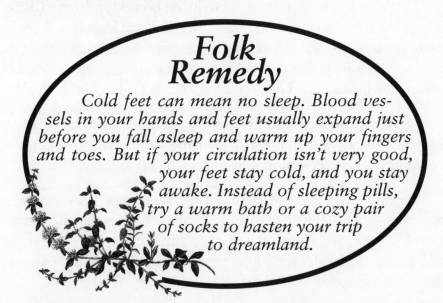

Folk Remedy

Cold feet can mean no sleep. Blood vessels in your hands and feet usually expand just before you fall asleep and warm up your fingers and toes. But if your circulation isn't very good, your feet stay cold, and you stay awake. Instead of sleeping pills, try a warm bath or a cozy pair of socks to hasten your trip to dreamland.

IRRITABLE BOWEL SYNDROME

Eliminate these IBS suspects

You've been looking forward to the neighborhood cookout all week. Then, suddenly, just as you're heading over with the potato salad, an attack of diarrhea forces you to spend the rest of the evening in your bathroom. It wouldn't be so bad if it only happened once in a blue moon, but this happens to you several times a week.

That's typical for a sufferer of irritable bowel syndrome (IBS), which is a group of symptoms, not a disease. If you have IBS, there is nothing physically wrong with your gastrointestinal tract, although you probably have symptoms like painful gas; bloating; and alternating constipation and diarrhea, which can lead to hemorrhoids.

People with IBS would like nothing better than to know what causes it and how to stop it. But instead of identifying one culprit, researchers keep finding new suspects to add to the lineup.

Sugar. Many people with bowel disorders have trouble absorbing lactose, fructose, and sorbitol. Lactose is the sugar found in milk, and fructose occurs naturally in fruit, corn syrup, and honey. Sorbitol, found in certain berries, is used as a sweetener in many foods.

Researchers in Israel wondered if eliminating these sweeteners from the diet could help people with bowel problems. They tested their theory by having IBS sufferers cut these sweeteners from their diets for one month. The results might motivate you to do the same. More than half of the study participants who returned for follow-up reported fewer IBS symptoms. The researchers concluded that people with IBS should try avoiding these sugars before opting for medicine. Try eliminating one type of sugar at a time to see if it helps you. Be sure to read labels carefully and consider visiting a nutritionist for advice.

Lack of sleep. New research shows that your IBS can be worse if you don't get enough sleep. In a two-month study, women with IBS reported worse symptoms following even one night of poor rest. Do whatever you must to get a good night's sleep. Unplug the phone, wear earplugs, or take a warm bath to help you settle down. Avoid caffeine and alcohol before bed — probably a good idea anyway if you have IBS — since these can interfere with your sleep. And shoot for eight hours of shut-eye every night.

Stress. Negative emotions, such as anger, sadness, and anxiety, can make IBS symptoms worse, and flare-ups are more likely when you're under stress. Concentrating on your breathing can be the key to learning to relax. Most people aren't aware of their breathing. After all, it's automatic. Check yourself during the day to see how you're doing. If you're taking shallow breaths from your chest, you need to take a minute to breathe slowly and deeply — as though you were breathing from your stomach. Concentrate on

---

What is it?

This common digestive disorder has no known cause or cure. With IBS, ordinary things cause your colon to overreact and spasm. These spasms can delay your stool, resulting in constipation; or they can speed things up, causing diarrhea. IBS isn't a life-threatening disease, but since it causes discomfort and anxiety, it can affect your quality of life.

Symptoms:
- Constipation
- Diarrhea
- Abdominal cramps and pain
- Gas
- Bloating

each breath until you feel yourself begin to relax. Do this several times each day until it's second nature to you.

You can also deal with negative emotions by learning to express yourself better. If you're someone who can never speak up, consider taking an assertiveness training class or asking a therapist to work with you so you'll gain confidence. Often, learning to express anger and other negative emotions leads to better health for IBS sufferers.

Foil IBS with antibiotics

Did you know you have microscopic bugs in your intestinal tract? Don't panic — everybody has them. In fact, you need a certain amount of these bugs, called bacteria, to process food and stay healthy. But sometimes they multiply to an unhealthy level, causing small intestinal bacterial overgrowth (SIBO).

On a hunch, researchers at Cedars-Sinai Medical Center in Los Angeles gave antibiotics to a group of people with irritable bowel syndrome (IBS). After 10 days, many of the people improved so much they no longer could be classified as IBS patients, and some were completely free of IBS. Dr. Henry C. Lin, senior author of the study and Director of the Cedars-Sinai GI Motility Program, thinks the study is significant for people with IBS.

"This is the first study," he says, "to demonstrate that complete eradication of SIBO with commonly prescribed antibiotics substantially improves the symptoms of IBS, especially those associated with bloating, diarrhea, and abdominal pain."

But because some of the people studied didn't respond to antibiotics, the researchers believe there must be other causes of IBS, too.

In order to be tested for SIBO, your doctor will likely want to give you a test called a lactulose hydrogen breath test or LHBT.

You'll have to fast overnight and then breathe into a machine that measures the amount of hydrogen your intestines make. If you're producing a large amount of hydrogen, you likely have an overgrowth of bacteria, and your doctor can prescribe an antibiotic.

Even if you aren't a good candidate for antibiotics, there are things you can do to keep the bacteria in your gut working for you.

Eat more yogurt. It sounds crazy, but eating more live bacteria can help keep your bowels healthier. The key is the type of bacteria you eat. Certain bacteria, like the ones in yogurt with active cultures, are friendly to your gut. Called probiotics, these help

Minimize bone loss in IBD

Inflammatory bowel disease (IBD), which includes Crohn's disease and ulcerative colitis, is much more serious than irritable bowel syndrome. If you have IBD, your intestines will show evidence of an actual disease process, and your doctor will likely prescribe medicine.

Recently, scientists discovered something new for people with IBD to watch for — osteoporosis.

Studies show IBD sufferers are 40 percent more likely to break their spine, hip, wrist, forearm, or a rib. Experts aren't sure why this is, but it might be due to prescribed drugs, or perhaps an inability to absorb enough nutrients.

More studies need to be done, but in the meantime, you can do everything possible to minimize bone loss. Eat plenty of calcium-rich foods, such as low-fat milk, yogurt, and Chinese cabbage. Drink calcium-fortified orange juice, so you can also load up on vitamin C, and eat plenty of bananas and other good sources of potassium. Buy fortified milk and get at least 15 minutes of sunshine every day so your skin can create vitamin D — critical for strong bones.

You can also fend off osteoporosis with weight-bearing exercises, so stay active. Even walking helps keep your bones strong.

restore the natural balance by keeping unfriendly bacteria at bay. Think of them as bacteria that fight on your side against bad bugs intent on taking over your small intestine. Yogurt with active cultures is an excellent source of probiotics. Try to eat yogurt without added sugar since many people with IBS also have trouble absorbing sugars. Check the label to make sure it says "active cultures." That means it was made with living bacteria. Yogurt made without live cultures won't do you much good.

Try supplements. You can also try probiotic supplements, such as acidophilus or lactobacillus capsules. You can find them wherever supplements are sold. These little capsules contain millions of good bacteria that can help restore balance to your gut. But don't forget to check the expiration date so you can be sure they're still alive.

Folk Remedy

To treat an upset stomach the way your great-grandmother might have done, use peppermint tea leaves from your local health food store. Pour one cup of boiling water over a heaping tablespoon of peppermint tea leaves and steep for five minutes. Drink a cup of this tea between meals, but no more than four cups a day.

Herbalists say menthol oil in the tea is responsible for the tummy-soothing effect. But don't give it to young children, because menthol can give them a choking feeling.

KIDNEY STONES

Action plan to prevent kidney stones

Think of kidney stones as a crime. To solve it, first you round up the usual suspects. These include two prime suspects — low fluid intake and a high-oxalate diet. If you don't get enough fluids, your urine becomes more concentrated, leading to crystals. Too many crystals can lead to stone formation. Foods high in oxalate include beets, rhubarb, strawberries, nuts, chocolate, spinach, and other green leafy vegetables. Other possible suspects include a low-calcium diet, which causes your body to absorb more oxalate, and a diet high in salt. Also take family history into account.

"The best advice is to maintain a high fluid intake, aiming for half water, with a goal of keeping very little color to the urine," says Dr. Richard W. Norman, professor and head of the urology department at Canada's Dalhousie University.

> ### What is it?
>
> These rock-like crystals form in your kidneys when chemicals in your urine build up to abnormal levels. Most kidney stones will pass out of your body by themselves, but since they can grow to be as big as golf balls and as jagged as glass, this can be quite painful.
>
> Symptoms:
> - Sharp, irregular pain in your lower back or side
> - Nausea and vomiting
> - Bloody, bad-smelling, or cloudy urine
> - Need to urinate often
> - Fever and chills
> - Weakness
> - Burning

But sometimes you have to sift through more evidence to solve a crime. Here are some more unusual strategies to stop kidney stones.

217

Switch sides. Avoiding kidney stones might be as simple as rolling over. Research by Dr. Marshall L. Stoller of the University of California at San Francisco shows that people who develop kidney stones on one side of the body also sleep on that side. He's not sure why, but theorizes it might have something to do with the change in blood flow to your kidneys caused by the sleeping position.

If you usually sleep on your right side, try sleeping on your left instead, and vice versa. You might get rid of those annoying stones. If you have trouble doing this, you can try the old tennis ball trick, a common way to stop snoring. Sew a tennis ball into the side of your pajamas, so you won't stay in that position. Or you can use a sleeping wedge to keep you facing the proper way during the night.

Trim the fat. Norman also explored the relationship between dietary fat and kidney stones. In one study, the link was stronger than anticipated. In other words, fat had a greater effect on kidney stones than was previously believed. However, in another study, he found no link at all between dietary fat and kidney stones.

"There is no association between dietary fat and risk of kidney stone formation in people with a normal gastrointestinal tract," Norman says, adding, "Diet should be one of moderation and variety."

You might not have to worry about kidney stones, but since fat contributes to so many health problems — like heart disease, stroke, diabetes, and cancer — it might be a good idea to limit your dietary fat anyway.

Pass on protein. A French study found that cutting your normal protein intake by about one-third can help protect against kidney stones. People in the study limited meat and fish to three servings a week and didn't have more than 100 grams of milk and cheese a day. Instead, they ate more pasta and rice.

To give you an idea of how little 100 grams is, consider this. A cup of skim milk is 245 grams, and a 1-ounce slice of mozzarella cheese is 28 grams.

"Protein intake increases urinary uric acid, which can increase stone risk through several mechanisms," Norman explains.

The goal is to keep your calories from animal protein at less than 10 percent of your total calories. Nonanimal sources of protein include beans, peas, seeds, and grains.

Go bananas. Simply getting the recommended dietary allowance (RDA) of potassium might not be good enough to prevent kidney stones. You need more, especially if your diet includes a lot of salt. A study from Brazil found that, although people ate plenty of potassium-rich foods and their total potassium intake fell within recommended levels, they still weren't getting enough potassium to combat kidney stones. Potassium helps by increasing the level of citrate in your urine.

Make an effort to eat more potassium-rich foods. These include bananas, tomatoes, oranges, avocados, figs, beans, and potatoes.

Tasty ways to 'liquidate' painful stones

Thirsty? If you want to combat kidney stones, you'd better be. Harvard studies show that the people who drink the most fluids have a better chance of avoiding these painful nuisances.

In one study, women who drank at least 11 8-ounce beverages a day were 38 percent less likely to develop kidney stones than women who drank less than six. Similar results were found in another study of men. The men who drank the most fluids had a 35 percent lower chance of getting kidney stones than those who drank the least.

But that's not the whole story. What beverage you choose also makes a difference. Here are the best — and worst — beverages to drink if you want to minimize your risk for kidney stones.

- **Coffee.** A piping hot cup of coffee might be just what you need to wake up — and bring down your chances of getting kidney stones by 10 percent. Like alcohol, caffeine waters down your urine and makes you go to the bathroom more often. That gives kidney stones little chance to develop. Oddly, decaf coffee also lowers your risk by 9 to 10 percent. This leads researchers to believe that something other than caffeine is at work.

- **Tea.** Even though tea was suspected to be high in oxalate, a substance that can contribute to kidney stones, the Harvard studies found that tea lowered men's kidney stone risk by 14 percent and women's risk by 8 percent. That's probably because very little of the harmful oxalate is absorbed by the body. Researchers figure the increased flow of diluted urine caused by the caffeine in tea counteracts the small increase in oxalate.

- **Lemonade.** This refreshing beverage contains a lot of citric acid, which is a part of citrate. Because citrate stops calcium-based stones from forming, one of the common causes of kidney stones is a lack of citrate in the urine. A University of California at San Francisco study tested lemonade on a small group of people with low levels of urinary citrate. Lemonade more than doubled the amount of citrate in the urine while also cutting down on the calcium. So next time you sip a cool glass of lemonade on a hot day, remember you're also putting kidney stones on ice.

Not all citrus fruits make good kidney stone-fighting drinks, however. Grapefruit juice actually increases your risk for kidney stones by as much as 44 percent. Researchers aren't sure why, but suspect that grapefruit juice might increase your body's absorption of oxalate from other foods. Another beverage you might want to avoid is apple juice, which increased men's risk for kidney stones by 35 percent but did not affect women's risk.

Wine and beer were actually the most effective beverages in preventing kidney stones in the Harvard studies. Alcohol likely helps fight kidney stones by making you urinate more often and by diluting your urine. However, alcohol contributes to so many health problems — including liver disease, pancreatitis, high blood pressure, and congestive heart failure — that it's not wise to take up drinking just to battle kidney stones. If you don't drink, don't start. If you do drink, limit your alcohol intake to one or two glasses of wine or beer a day.

LACTOSE INTOLERANCE

Look out for lactose tricks and traps

If you think you're lactose intolerant, think again. Even if you have the nausea, cramps, diarrhea, and bloating that normally come with this condition, you might actually suffer from another problem entirely.

Rule out other causes. Before you take any drastic steps, make sure you really are lactose intolerant. Other sugars besides lactose sometimes cause the same unpleasant reactions.

Your problem could stem from fructose, found naturally in honey, figs, pears, prunes, and grapes. It's also used in corn syrup to sweeten foods, gums, candies, and sodas. Other culprits include sorbitol, mannitol, and xylitol, which are in sugarless or diet foods, beverages, and gums.

Many people have trouble absorbing these substances. If you eat too much of these foods, the non-absorbed sugars move into the large intestine and cause the same problems as lactose intolerance.

Don't forget about gluten, either. This protein in wheat, rye, barley, and oats gives a lot of people trouble. You could just be sensitive to gluten or have celiac disease, in which case gluten actually damages your intestines. You'd experience weight loss, bloating, gas, weakness, and changes in your bowel habits. If you have celiac disease, you must completely avoid foods containing gluten. You'll have to read labels carefully since gluten pops up in all sorts of unexpected places — even ice cream.

Keep a food diary so you can pinpoint which foods cause which symptoms. This will help your doctor determine your problem.

Beware of hidden lactose. Like gluten, lactose crops up in some unlikely places. If you are lactose intolerant, you have to be very alert.

For example, whey, the watery liquid that's left when milk becomes cheese, is in processed foods like crackers. And it contains lactose. So does dry, or powdered, milk. Perhaps most alarming is that about 20 percent of all prescription drugs and 6 percent of all over-the-counter products contain lactose.

Make sure you read all food and drug labels very carefully, and ask your pharmacist about any medication you're not sure of.

But even careful attention to labels can't entirely protect you. According to *FDA Consumer* magazine, current labeling guidelines leave some loopholes. Manufacturers can use the term "nondairy" even when the product contains milk byproducts. And there are more than a dozen ways to include milk protein in the list of ingredients without actually using the word "milk."

If you are particularly intolerant, it might be a good idea to limit your processed foods, and avoid anything with unfamiliar ingredients.

> ### *What is it?*
> Lactose intolerance is another way to say you have trouble digesting milk and other dairy products. This happens when your small intestine doesn't produce enough of the special enzyme that breaks down lactose, the main sugar in dairy foods.
>
> Symptoms:
> - Nausea
> - Gas
> - Diarrhea
> - Bloating
> - Cramps

Become creative. Don't let lactose intolerance stop you from enjoying food. Try making some substitutions in your recipes. For example, if something calls for dry milk, try using the same amount of water instead. Experiment. You might find some interesting — and tasty — solutions.

It's possible you can dabble in dairy products now and then. While some people — often those of Asian or African descent — are very sensitive and must avoid all lactose, others can eat a small amount. Know your limit, and make sure your menu doesn't go over it.

Solve your dairy dilemma

Gas pains again? Don't despair if you're a dairy lover who's lactose intolerant. You may not have to give up milk products altogether to avoid those painful digestive problems. Different people can handle different amounts of lactose. So, while milk or cheese may give you grief, yogurt might not be a problem. Experiment with one type of dairy food at a time to determine what you can eat and what you need to steer clear of.

For the growing numbers of lactose-intolerant people, most grocery stores now carry products to help solve your dairy dilemma. Lactose-reduced milk and cheese are easy to find. You can even buy lactase enzymes to help you digest foods more easily.

You should be able to work some dairy into your diet, but if you're cutting back, be sure to get enough calcium. Good nondairy sources include kale, sardines, turnip greens, salmon, peanuts, and pinto beans.

MEMORY LOSS

Helpful hints to mend your memory

Once upon a time, you could rattle off birthdays, phone numbers, and addresses, keep track of appointments without using a date book, and remember every funny story from your childhood.

Now, you're lucky if you remember what you ate for lunch. If your memory batteries seem to be running low, try these tips for recharging them.

Aim for more antioxidants. Many foods contain naturally occurring chemicals that fight damaging free radicals in your body. Beta carotene, which your body converts to vitamin A, is one of these antioxidants. By protecting your brain cells, beta carotene helps you think, reason, and remember. Unfortunately, millions of people throughout the world don't get enough vitamin A. Even just one milligram of beta carotene a day makes a big difference. Carrots, sweet potatoes, apricots, tomatoes, broccoli, cantaloupe, and collard greens are all good sources.

Vitamins C and E also fight free radical damage and poor memory. In fact, vitamin E might help ward off Alzheimer's. Look for vitamin C in oranges, grapefruit, broccoli,

---

What is it?

Sometimes you simply can't remember things. Maybe it's trouble recalling a recent event, finding where you placed an object, or putting a name to a face or place.

Occasional memory loss is a normal part of brain aging. But when it becomes a frequent and noticeable problem, it could signal a much more serious condition, like Alzheimer's disease or another form of dementia.

Symptoms:
↝ Forgetfulness
↝ Confusion

peppers, cantaloupe, and strawberries. You can find vitamin E in wheat germ, nuts, seeds, and vegetable oils.

Gather memories with herbs. Ginkgo and ginseng both boost memory and concentration. They also fight stress and anxiety and give you energy.

In clinical studies, ginkgo increased blood flow to the brain by 70 percent in seniors. That means more brainpower and better short-term memory. This ancient herb also helps fight absent-mindedness, confusion, tiredness, depression, dizziness, tinnitus, and headaches — all signs of dementia. Look for pure ginkgo biloba extract (GBE or GBX), and take 40 milligrams three times a day. Be patient; it might be a few weeks before you notice results.

To get the benefits of ginseng, chew on ginseng roots or make tea from a small chunk of root. You can also buy a variety of ginseng products, including teas, capsules, extracts, tablets, wine, chewing gum, cola, and candy. Read their labels to make sure they contain between 4 and 7 percent ginsenosides, the steroid-like compounds found in the bark or outer layer of the root.

Give your mind a workout. Read, solve a crossword puzzle, take night classes, or find new hobbies. Just keep your mind challenged. Your brain needs to stay in shape to perform at its best. Vary your activities to maximize your brainpower.

Sip, slurp, and swallow. Just because you're confused or show other signs of dementia doesn't mean you have Alzheimer's disease. It might mean you simply need to drink more water. Dehydration causes confusion, disorientation, and other problems. Drink water even if you're not thirsty.

Beef up your B's. Folate, thiamin, B6, and B12 are B vitamins that play key roles in brain function. No wonder people with chronic B deficiencies score lower on memory and problem solving tests, while those receiving a boost of B vitamins perform better. A shortage of B vitamins may even lead to Alzheimer's. For folate, eat spinach, beets, avocados, asparagus, and other vegetables. Low-fat cheese, fish, and poultry supply you with B12, and potatoes, beans, and watermelon provide B6 and thiamin.

Break those bad habits. Smokers and heavy drinkers already have plenty of health risks. Add memory loss to the list. A recent study of 3,000 elderly men showed that those who smoked throughout their middle years were one-third more likely to have memory loss than men who had never smoked. Even those who once smoked but quit had some memory loss. In addition, alcohol kills brain cells, and drinking heavily (more than two drinks a day) reduces blood flow to the part of the brain that makes memories.

Get your forty winks. Sleeping is a natural way to boost mind-improving hormones. Not getting enough sleep harms your ability to store information in your long-term memory. Aim for a regular sleep routine, where you go to bed and wake up at the same time every day.

Start the day off right. Breakfast gives your brain the fuel it needs for the day. When you wake up, help yourself to a bowl of cereal or a bagel. Studies show children who eat breakfast do better on tests than those who skip this important meal. Other studies suggest something sugary — like certain cereals or orange juice — gives your brain a boost. But don't go overboard. Just a little of the sweet stuff keeps your brain charged all day.

Check those medications. Your memory loss may not have anything to do with you. It could be a side effect of your prescription drugs. Ask your doctor about switching to a different medication.

Lubricate your brain. In an Italian study of nearly 300 seniors, those who ate at least 5 tablespoons of olive oil a day tested best on memory and problem solving skills. It's the monounsaturated fat that enhances your brainpower, but olive oil also has vitamin E and other antioxidants. Next time you're in the kitchen, pour on the olive oil instead of corn or soybean oils.

Beware of ginkgo's dark side

There's potential danger hidden among the benefits of ginkgo biloba. This popular memory-boosting herb might cause seizures.

Seven incidents have been reported to the FDA's special division that tracks illness or injury from dietary supplements. Three of these incidents involved ginkgo biloba itself, while the other four involved products with ginkgo biloba as an ingredient. Events ranged from "epileptic-type seizures" to "seizure and stroke" to "cardiac arrest and seizure."

Experts don't know why ginkgo caused seizures in these cases. However, products containing ginkgo seeds, as opposed to ginkgo leaf extract, have been linked to seizures in the past. So, one explanation is that ginkgo seeds contaminated these ginkgo products.

If you are prone to seizures or taking medication that lists seizures as a possible side effect, talk to your doctor before taking ginkgo.

Iron out your wrinkled memory. Poor memory could be a sign of iron deficiency, especially if you also look pale and feel sad and tired. If you're a vegetarian or regularly take nonsteroidal anti-inflammatory drugs (NSAIDs), you may not be getting enough iron. Even though you find iron mostly in meat, you can also get it from legumes and green leafy vegetables.

Tackle forgetfulness with technology

Take advantage of the marvels of modern technology for help with a faltering memory. Lots of gee-whiz gizmos can lend a hand in remembering to take pills, make appointments, and keep in touch with friends.

- ✤ **Personal Digital Assistant (PDA).** The latest in computer wizardry, a PDA can keep track of phone numbers, addresses, appointments, and anything else your busy schedule calls for.

- ✦ **Portable alarm clock and wristwatches.** They ring, buzz, vibrate, and even talk. Simply set an alarm and you may never forget a thing again. Look for brands that have a multiple alarm feature and an automatic reset timer.

- ✦ **Automatic pill dispenser.** Program these wonder machines to release your pills at specific times during the day.

- ✦ **Telephones.** All sorts of nifty phones are on the market. One dials a number when you say the name of the person you want to call and another has a place for photographs so you can easily put a phone number with a face.

Talk with your doctor about your specific needs, then contact these companies for a full catalog of their products:

Dynamic Living
1265 John Fitch Blvd. #9
South Windsor, CT 06074
888-940-0605
<www.dynamic-living.com>

MaxiAids, Inc
42 Executive Blvd.
Farmingdale, NY 11735
800-522-6294
<www.maxiaids.com>

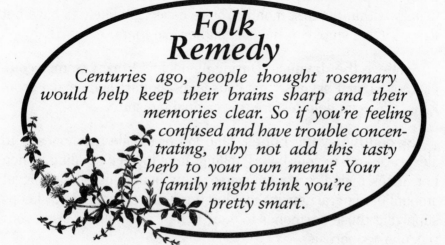

Folk Remedy

Centuries ago, people thought rosemary would help keep their brains sharp and their memories clear. So if you're feeling confused and have trouble concentrating, why not add this tasty herb to your own menu? Your family might think you're pretty smart.

MENOPAUSE

Startling pros and cons of HRT

It's true that hormones can help relieve symptoms of menopause — hot flashes, dry skin, and fatigue — but at what price? Hormone replacement therapy (HRT) has come under fire lately for some worrisome side effects. Yet thousands of women swear by and depend on the benefits.

Study the following pros and cons, and talk to your doctor so you can make an informed decision.

Lower the heat. Because estrogen is involved in regulating your body temperature, without it, your body acts like a house with a broken thermostat. Not enough estrogen means hot flashes. HRT can help bring your estrogen levels — and your skin temperature — back in line. In fact, it could eliminate your hot flashes, usually within the first month. You're especially likely to have hot flashes if you smoke, or if your mother had them.

Relieve the dryness. During menopause, many women complain of vaginal dryness that causes discomfort and sexual problems. HRT can help restore this vaginal moisture.

Strengthen your bones. One job of female hormones is to alert receptors in your bones, telling them to keep building. When hormones dwindle at menopause, your bones lose a significant amount of mineral density, making them more fragile. HRT keeps supplying those hormones to your bones, and so decreases your risk of osteoporosis.

Stay sharp. When estrogen levels start tapering off in midlife, many women report having trouble concentrating and remembering details. A recent study found that dementia developed more often in women with low estrogen levels. Since HRT provides your body with regular doses of estrogen, it might help you think more clearly and avoid dementia. Some researchers think it could even help prevent degenerative brain diseases such as Alzheimer's.

Hold down the pressure. Menopause often means an increase in blood pressure. But, again, estrogen comes to the rescue. Contrary to popular thought, HRT does not increase blood pressure. Rather, transdermal, or patch, estrogen can lower blood pressure — although oral estrogen has no effect. Talk to your doctor about your specific health needs.

Rest easier. The University of Toronto and St. Michael's Hospital Sleep Laboratory tried to clear up the relationship between sleep apnea — a condition that causes you to stop breathing while sleeping — and menopause.

They found twice as many women past menopause suffer from sleep apnea as pre-menopausal women. And it has more to do with estrogen levels than the traditional causes of the disorder, like weight and neck size. Since being post-menopausal increases your risk of suffering from sleep apnea, HRT could be one way to fight this serious breathing disorder.

What is it?

Known as the "change of life," menopause occurs when a woman permanently stops menstruating and her ovaries produce less and less estrogen and progesterone. This process is very gradual, sometimes lasting for several years. When you haven't had your period for one whole year, then you have reached the final stage of menopause.

Symptoms:
- Missed periods
- Hot flashes and sweating
- Vaginal dryness
- Urinary tract or vaginal infections

Save your knees. Osteoarthritis, a form of arthritis where joint cartilage wears away, is a particular threat to older women. And since research shows estrogen plays a role in the structure of normal joints, experts believe estrogen therapy could protect you from this major cause of disability after menopause. It's a fact, taking estrogen replacement therapy (ERT) for more than five years has been linked to more and stronger knee cartilage.

Dishearten your heart. If you're one of many women with a history of heart disease, there's disturbing news.

Lori Mosca, M.D., Ph.D., director of preventive cardiology at New York Presbyterian Hospital of Columbia and Cornell Universities, says, "For many years, cardiologists and other health care providers who take care of women have assumed that HRT protects the heart. But at this time there is not sufficient evidence to make that claim."

Even the American Heart Association no longer supports starting HRT solely to prevent heart attacks and strokes. New studies reveal that, at least in the first year of hormone therapy, your risk of heart problems actually goes up.

Hinder your breathing. HRT can make airway inflammation or spasms worse. That will increase your risk of developing asthma — by as much as 80 percent, according to the well known Nurses' Health Study. Your risk grows according to how much and how long you take estrogen.

Endure break-through bleeding. As you probably know, HRT can cause occasional, light uterine bleeding. Although unpredictable and a nuisance, it's not considered a medical problem.

Complicate mammograms. It's not permanent, but while you're on HRT, your breast tissue will probably change — becoming more compact or dense. This makes it hard for radiologists to read your mammograms and can affect how accurately you're screened for breast cancer. Once you stop using HRT, your breasts should return to normal.

Realize a cancer risk. If you take estrogen for 10 years or more after menopause, your chances of getting — and dying from

— ovarian cancer increase. No one can explain exactly why. Experts do know, however, taking estrogen for less than 10 years won't significantly raise your risk. There's also no information on the risk for women taking estrogen combined with progestin.

Another, more rare, type of cancer is on the rise in women over 50. Lobular carcinoma affects the small spaces in your breasts that contain milk-producing glands. While some experts believe HRT is associated with this cancer, there's not yet enough hard evidence.

Go up against gallstones. Women taking estrogen replacement therapy are at higher risk for developing gallstones. One study found those with heart disease taking HRT were 40 percent more likely to develop gallbladder disease. Talk to your doctor about switching to patch estrogen or even a different kind of oral estrogen. Sometimes this is enough to decrease side effects.

Master midlife weight gain

You're not destined to jump three dress sizes just because you're going through menopause. With a little work, you can hold the scales steady during this time of change — even lose weight.

Most women gain an average of one pound per year during menopause. But by cutting calories, avoiding saturated fat, and exercising in your spare time, you can not only keep from gaining weight, but may actually drop a few pounds.

While weight control is important, other equally valuable health benefits can come from these lifestyle changes. You'll impact your blood pressure, and insulin, cholesterol, and triglyceride levels.

You too can stay fit through menopause and beyond. Think of dieting and exercising as a way of pampering yourself during this important time of your life. For moral support, join other women who have similar goals. Look for an aerobics or dance class, a swimming group, or walking club.

Nature manages menopause

There are many reasons why you would turn to herbs and nutrients to combat the symptoms of menopause. Perhaps hormone therapy is simply wrong for you — physically or emotionally. Sit down with your doctor and honestly assess your overall health, your risk for osteoporosis and heart disease, and the pros and cons of aggressive drugs. Then explore alternative therapies that are, after all, the source of many traditional medications.

Cool down with cohosh. If hot flashes and mood swings are bothering you, black cohosh could be just the thing you need. Once called squaw root, Native Americans used this plant for thousands of years to treat female problems.

Today, doctors in Germany often prescribe black cohosh to treat PMS symptoms as well as anxiety, mild depression, and sweating in menopausal women. The plant has an estrogen-like effect, and reduces levels of a hormone that causes hot flashes.

You'll find it in capsules where supplements are sold. Try taking 40 milligrams (mg) a day, but not for longer than six months.

Rely on St. John. Hippocrates, of ancient Greece, recommended the popular herb St. John's wort for menstrual problems. Over two thousand years later, menopausal women still use it to feel better physically and sexually. Best of all, it comes with very few side effects. Although you may have to stay out of strong sun to avoid a rash, people rarely show allergic reactions.

Be sure the supplement you buy is a reputable brand and contains 0.3 percent hypericin, the active ingredient. The usual dosage is 300 mg, three times daily. Talk to your doctor about using St. John's wort for longer than a few weeks.

Add vitamin A. Most women over 50 need 4,000 IU (international units) or 800 RE (retinol equivalents) of vitamin A every

Don't blame menopause for sinking sex life

Has your sex life been in the doldrums since you crossed the threshold of menopause? Before you jump to any conclusions, consider this.

Experts studied the sexual functioning of 200 women going through menopause (but not on hormone replacement therapy). As expected, menopause was related to a decrease in sexual desire and arousal compared to when the women were younger.

But the story doesn't end there. When the women were questioned more closely, it turned out other factors had an even bigger effect on their sex life than menopause.

Having a new partner, their physical and mental health, and whether or not they smoked were all more important to sexual functioning than being menopausal.

Instead of resigning yourself to fizzle instead of fireworks, look carefully at your life for clues. Could you be suffering from low-grade depression? Are you still smoking? Do you have health problems that are robbing you of energy? Focusing on these factors and getting help for them could put you back on the road to sexual satisfaction.

day. You get it naturally in the form of beta carotene in foods. Dark green and yellow-orange vegetables are good sources.

During menopause, vitamin A can help counteract dry skin and fight bothersome yeast infections. Also a powerful antioxidant, it helps prevent cancer.

Build up your Bs. Vitamins B2, B6, and B12 are water-soluble vitamins your body flushes out daily. That means you need to replace them often. They help you turn food into energy; fight migraines, osteoporosis, and depression; and keep your heart healthy. Eat liver, mushrooms, whole grains, bananas, nuts, seeds, eggs, fish, and cauliflower.

Depend on E. Don't let heart disease sneak up on you in middle age as it does for many women. Vitamin E works like an antioxidant to keep cholesterol from damaging your arteries. It can also reduce hot flashes and keep your skin soft and younger looking. Add E to your diet with nuts, seeds, avocados, canola oil, and low-fat creamy salad dressings.

Count on calcium. Some experts see a connection between low calcium and hot flashes. So, a glass of skim milk might keep you feeling cool long after you drink it. In addition, calcium is important for strong bones — a major concern during menopause. Eat yogurt, cheese, spinach, beans, Chinese cabbage, seeds, and almonds.

Study the soy issue. When menopause steals your estrogen, replace it with plant sources. Also called phytoestrogens, these can give you some of the protective benefits of natural estrogen. Soy-based foods, like soybeans, tofu, miso, and soy nuts, seem to help many women.

However, experts have concerns. Although some research shows soy improves thinking, helps your heart, and prevents osteoporosis, others suggest it makes your brain age faster. The latest buzz is the more soy you eat, the greater your risk of developing senility.

Talk to your doctor about eating soy during menopause. Because it comes from a bean, you might feel a bit gassy at first, so add it to your diet gradually. And, as in most things in life, moderation is best.

You can find out more about living an all-natural menopause by consulting a naturopathic physician (ND). These doctors specialize in alternative treatments — no drugs or surgeries. To find an

ND near you, go to the Worldwide Directory of Naturopathic Practitioners, Colleges, and Organizations on the Internet at <www.naturopathics.com>. Or contact:

The American Association of Naturopathic Physicians
8201 Greensboro Drive, Suite 300
McLean, VA 2210
703-610-9037

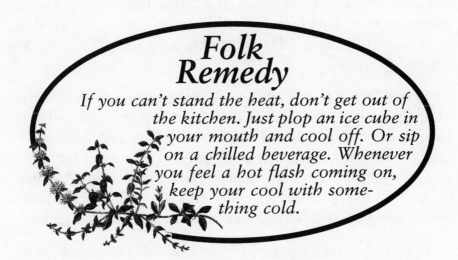

Folk Remedy

If you can't stand the heat, don't get out of the kitchen. Just plop an ice cube in your mouth and cool off. Or sip on a chilled beverage. Whenever you feel a hot flash coming on, keep your cool with something cold.

MUSCLE PAIN

6 amazing ways to avoid muscle pain

Hollering "Fore!" before teeing off does not count as a warm-up exercise. Unfortunately, most recreational golfers don't do much more than that.

Golf may seem like a calm, relaxing, low-risk activity, but you still need to warm up properly to avoid muscle pain. A recent Australian study found that half of all golfers don't warm up at all before hitting the links. Of those who do, most just take a few practice swings.

In fact, less than 3 percent of golfers go through an effective warm-up routine. This involves a few brief aerobic exercises to get your blood flowing, followed by stretching "the golf muscles" — hands, wrists, forearms, shoulders, lower back, chest, trunk, hamstrings, and groin. After stretching, practice your swing, building up gradually to big, powerful strokes. This approach might do more than protect you from injury — it could also improve your game.

Of course, preventing muscle pain is not limited to golf. In all aspects of everyday life, you can take steps to avoid aching muscles.

Stand up straight. Poor posture can lead to back pain and a host of other physical problems. That's because slouching, slumping, and sitting around too much puts extra strain on your muscles. Rounded shoulders and a noticeable curve in your lower back are telltale signs of poor posture. You can check your posture

— and improve it — by either standing or sitting against a wall. With your shoulders and upper back touching the wall, raise your arms over your head and try to touch the wall. If you can do this easily, you have good posture. If not, keep trying. You'll strengthen your back and shoulder muscles and straighten out your spine. Yoga and tai chi can also help improve your posture.

Work out wisely. You're less likely to injure your muscles if you get in the habit of using them. A regular exercise routine helps tremendously. Come up with a schedule that features both aerobic and weight training exercises. Aerobic activities, like walking, jogging, biking, or swimming, help you lose weight and improve circulation, while weight lifting builds strength and guards your muscles from injury. You also build greater support for your spine, which leads to better posture and less back pain. If you're not used to being active, ease into an exercise program gradually.

> ### *What is it?*
> It could be a dull ache or a throbbing agony. You may call it a "charley horse," a strain, a cramp, a spasm, or a tear. But no matter what its description, a variety of things cause muscle pain — overuse, dehydration, heat, cold, or even a more serious condition that requires medical help.
>
> Symptoms:
> ⤙ Tenderness, cramps, or soreness
> ⤙ General muscle weakness
> ⤙ Fatigue

Loosen up. Before and after your workouts, take some time to stretch. Stretching improves your flexibility and prevents your muscles from tightening up and causing injury. You can also stretch in between workouts anytime. It's a great way to keep your muscles limber. Here's a quick rundown of some areas to stretch and how to stretch them.

⤙ **Calves.** Stand with one leg bent and one leg straight back. Keep your back straight and slowly move your front foot forward. You'll feel a pull in the calf muscle in your back leg. Hold for 10 to 20 seconds. Do it again, then switch legs.

◈ **Shoulders and upper back.** Clasp your hands behind and above your head. Press your shoulders and elbows back for 10 to 20 seconds.

◈ **Groin.** Stand with your feet wide apart and your hands on your hips. Bend one leg while keeping your weight over the straight leg. You'll feel a pull in the groin muscle of your straight leg. Hold for 10 to 20 seconds. Repeat and switch legs.

◈ **Sides.** Clasp your hands high above your head. Lean sideways until you feel a pull in your side. Hold for 10 to 20 seconds. Do this a few more times before leaning to the other side.

◈ **Hips and back.** Clasp your hands in front of you and rotate as far as you can to the right. Hold for 10 to 20 seconds and repeat this exercise five times before doing the same thing to the left.

◈ **Quadriceps.** Stand on your right leg. With your left hand, take hold of your left foot and pull your knee back. You'll feel a pull in the front of your thigh. Hold for 10 to 20 seconds, then repeat and switch legs.

◈ **Hamstrings.** Stand with your feet wide apart. Push your rear end back a bit and bend forward, with your hands stretching toward a spot on the ground well in front of your feet. You'll feel it in the backs of your thighs. Hold for 10 to 20 seconds. As you get more flexible, you can do this exercise with your feet closer together.

Find your fit. One size does not always fit all. No matter what you're doing, make sure you use the proper size equipment, including shoes. Your body has its own distinct shape. Forcing it to adapt to someone else's could result in strained muscles. This applies to car seats and computer keyboards, as well as sporting equipment. Also make sure you use the proper technique. The best equipment in the world is no good if you don't use it right.

Shed that spare tire. The flab around your middle that comes with aging already ruined your figure. Now it might also ruin your back. In a recent Japanese study, women who had chronic low back pain were bigger around the middle than women without back pain. Try to lose some weight and strengthen the muscles in your legs to take some of the strain off your back. Strengthening your abdomen will also benefit your back, because your stomach muscles help support your spine.

Rest when it's best. Know the difference between a healthy tiredness and fatigue. You might feel tired after a good, long workout, but don't overdo your training. Too much activity causes a buildup of waste products in your body and wears out your muscles. Fatigue can be serious and require up to three weeks of complete rest.

Pulverize pain with these proven tips

Over 80 percent of people experience back pain at one time or another. Sadly, most people suffer when they don't have to. Instead of popping painkillers that could have dangerous side effects, turn to these natural ways to relieve your pain.

Get your blood flowing. Soaking your feet in lavender could work wonders on your tense muscles. The lavender gets blood flowing all over your body — like an internal hot compress — and that's exactly what your muscles need for fast healing.

Just sit in your favorite chair, pull up a basin, and fill it with hot, but not scalding, water. For every quart of water in the basin, pour in five to 10 drops of lavender essential oil. Stir the water before putting your feet in, and soak for at least 10 minutes.

Massage pain away. Science has finally shown what most people have known for years — a good massage works wonders for muscle pain. Your best bet is to make an appointment with a massage professional. But if you want immediate relief, ask a friend or loved one to give you a massage using this essential oil potion:

> 12 drops of lavender oil
> 6 drops of rosemary oil
> 4 drops of juniper oil
> 3 drops of peppermint oil

Mix the essential oils in an amber glass bottle and then add one tablespoon of vegetable oil and one tablespoon of a carrier oil, like sweet almond or apricot kernel. Stir and rub into your sore muscles.

Soak in a spa. Massaging water jets, steamy hot water, soothing support — these are the three main reasons experts suggest taking a dip in a whirlpool or spa. The hot water in the pool dilates, or opens up, your blood vessels, allowing more blood to flow to your muscles. The water also supports your sore muscles and joints, making it easier to do strengthening exercises and stretches. Plus, the jet nozzles push out water and air at just the right pressure, kneading and relaxing your muscles.

Ease your emotions. You've heard anger can lead to heart attacks, but back pain? That's right. Scientific research has confirmed that negative emotions — like anger and anxiety — could cause your sensations of pain to be stronger than they normally would. Holding in these emotions could make it even worse. Positive emotions — even fear, which in time of danger is positive — appear to make you less susceptible to pain.

Attain the unthinkable with yoga. If you want to take fewer painkillers and still feel better, try yoga. Volunteers in a cutting-edge study from the University of California at Los Angeles did just that. They did yoga exercises, a mix of breathing control and stretching, three times a week for four weeks. Each session only took an hour and a half.

Try these yoga exercises to see if it's for you.

- **Cat breath.** Get on your hands and knees while looking straight ahead. Breathe in, arch your back a little, and hold for three seconds. Then, breathe out, round your back up, and suck your stomach in. Tuck your chin in and hold for another three.

- **Knee squeeze.** Lie on your back with your arms on the ground over your head. Bend your left knee up, lift your head toward it, and wrap your arms around your knee. Hold your breath and pull your knee to your chest for three seconds. Breathe out, lower your leg and arms, and do the same thing with your right knee. Do it three times for each leg, then three times with both legs.

To find out more about yoga, visit your local fitness center, recreation department, or YMCA to see if they offer classes. Most important, always talk with your doctor before you start any new exercise routine.

Try an herbal painkiller. Almost 76,000 people each year rush to the hospital because of the side effects of their non-steroidal anti-inflammatory drugs (NSAIDs). One-tenth of these people die — and that's in the United States alone. There is a solution to this problem — herbal painkillers. They could put an end to your pain without dangerous side effects.

- **Cramp bark.** Great for weekend warriors, this herb relaxes strained muscles. Herbal experts suggest boiling one teaspoon of the bark in one cup of water, then straining and drinking this concoction three times a day. Cramp bark is also available as a lotion.

- **Valerian.** If you know you're about to meet stress head on, take these supplements according to the directions on the pack. Valerian could help soothe your mind before your muscles tense up.

➤ **Willow bark.** In a recent study, almost 40 percent of the participants taking willow bark extract were amazed when the herb swept away their pain. They took 240 milligrams for only four weeks. The ingredient in willow bark that makes it such a powerful painkiller is salicylate, the same active ingredient in aspirin.

Speed recovery of sore muscles

Do you want something that could ease muscle inflammation and soreness just as well as aspirin and other over-the-counter medications — without harsh side effects? The solution might be as close as your kitchen. Rely on these remedies to fend off everyday muscle soreness, like after a workout. Or use them for more serious injuries, like strains, tears, and chronic back pain.

Turn to vitamin C. Your muscles might be crying out for vitamin C if you have aches, pains, or swelling after a workout. This superstar of the vitamin world helps produce and maintain collagen, a protein that builds and repairs cartilage, ligaments, muscles, bones, and anything else that holds you together. As a champion antioxidant, vitamin C also has the power to help when your muscles are injured or inflamed. That's when infection and your body's natural healing process cause free radicals to build up in the damaged tissue. These renegade chemicals can cause even more harm to your body unless, of course, you send in vitamin C to take care of them.

Some experts suggest taking 500 milligrams (mg) of vitamin C ur times a day when you have swollen or injured muscles. To vent everyday soreness, take 500 mg before you hit the gym, pool, or the track.

ave a snack. Eat a turkey sandwich after you work out if nt your muscles to recover and heal faster. That way, you'll a rich source of leucine, an essential amino acid. Amino acids are the building blocks of protein, and leucine appears to be the one in charge of building muscle protein. To get more out of this important muscle fuel:

- Eat some lean meat, dairy foods, or a protein bar right after — not before or during — your workout. These foods, as well as some sports drinks, are good sources of leucine.

- Wash your snack down with a carbohydrate-rich fluid, like juice or a sports drink.

- Maintain a balanced diet, with protein making up 30 percent of your total calories.

Cut out caffeine. If you suffer from a backache or other chronic pain, consider cutting coffee and soft drinks from your diet. They are the top two sources of caffeine, and caffeine could be preventing your body's natural pain fighters from doing their job. It does this by lowering levels of "feel good" chemicals called endorphins and by boosting levels of epinephrine, a compound that can make your muscle nerves more sensitive to pain. On top of this, caffeine flushes calcium out of your body, lowering the mineral content of your bones and making them more prone to microfractures. These tiny breaks in your vertebrae, over time, can cause a big pain in your back.

Your best bet is to back off the caffeine and see if it helps. This doesn't seem to work for everyone. In fact, caffeine actually helps some people deal with pain. That's why it's an ingredient in many over-the-counter pain relievers.

Keep some mustard handy. A squirt of mustard and a cup of water are all you need to stop a muscle cramp in its tracks, according to the trainers at the University of Alabama. They say it works wonders for their star athletes. Though researchers haven't studied mustard's cramp-relieving power, they think vinegar is the ingredient responsible. The next time you're working out, bring along a few packets of mustard. When a cramp strikes, slurp down the contents of one package with some water. Repeat every two minutes until the mustard turns the tide against your cramps.

Drink more water. Dehydration is probably the most common cause of muscle cramps — and the easiest to prevent. Drink at least eight glasses of water each day to wash away painful cramps before they start.

Mind your minerals. Drinking water might not be enough to stop cramps if you're already dehydrated. You'll need healthy foods, too. That's because you could also be low in important minerals, like

The latest twist on back pain

Your back brace might not protect you from injury when you're lugging something heavy, according to recent research from the Centers for Disease Control and Prevention (CDC). The researchers backed their findings with two years of research on over 6,300 people, who all had jobs involving backbreaking labor. The workers who wore braces experienced just as many back problems as workers who didn't wear them.

Since past studies have shown that braces might help, these findings are controversial. So if you feel safer with a back brace, wear it.

Whether you wear a brace or not, the experts suggest following these do's and don'ts when you're lifting to prevent painful injuries:

- ✎ Do bend at the knees and the hips.
- ✎ Don't bend at the waist.
- ✎ Do keep your back straight.
- ✎ Don't twist your back into an awkward position.
- ✎ Do lift with your legs and pull the object close to you with your arms.
- ✎ Don't reach for or try to lift objects above shoulder height.

potassium, magnesium, and calcium — and plain old water won't replenish these. For more potassium, eat bananas, dried apricots, figs, or a ripe avocado. Try eating almonds, cashews, apricots, whole grains, or greens to raise your magnesium level. And dairy products, turnip greens, sardines, and oysters are great sources of calcium.

Get a leg up with quinine. Taking the edge off nighttime leg cramps could be as simple as drinking a cup (8 ounces) of tonic water. The fizzy drink contains almost 30 mg of quinine, which could be enough to get the job done. Try spritzing it with lemon or orange juice to zip up the flavor. But be careful — too much quinine can cause serious side effects. So if one cup of tonic doesn't work, move on to another remedy.

Baby your back with the perfect mattress

In the United States alone, over 40 million adults suffer from lower back pain. And more than 50 percent of them lose a good night's sleep because of it. The difference between these insomniacs and the back pain sufferers who sleep well could be their mattresses. A bad mattress can throw your spine out of whack and put stress on the muscles, ligaments, and nerves in your back. That leaves you tossing and turning all night.

To put an end to this agony, it's important to know when to ditch your old mattress and spring for a new one. Here's how you can decide what's best for you.

Know when to say when. According to Nancy Butler of the Better Sleep Council, your mattress might be worn out without you knowing it. Most mattresses can last over 10 years, but depending on the brand and how much daily wear and tear you put on it, you might need a new one well before then.

"Mattresses wear out gradually," Butler explains, so it's hard to tell exactly when it goes. After a while, she warns, "a mattress loses its support, but it still feels familiar to you." That's why it's important to be wary of the warning signs of a bad mattress. "There are four things we tell people to look for," Butler says. Being achy and stiff in the morning is the first sign. Also, take note if you're not getting as good a slumber as you were a year ago. If the last good night's rest you had took place in a hotel bed or somewhere other than your own bedroom, that's a good indication. Lastly, if your mattress starts showing its age — torn fabric, sagging middle, creaking springs — then you know it's "very far gone."

Check underneath the bed. No, not for monsters, but for your box spring. It's important to make sure it's in good shape, too. Your mattress and your box spring work together to give you a good night's sleep. So if you buy a new mattress, you probably will need to buy a new box spring as well.

Give your mattress a second life. You might not need to buy anything. If your mattress and your box spring are still in good shape — but your mattress is just too hard for your liking — look into buying a foam roll or a feather bed to lay on top of it. They'll provide an extra cushion that could make all the difference between counting sheep and deep sleep.

Supersize your mattress. If you and your spouse get in each other's hair during the night, a bigger mattress could be all you need. Experts suggest upsizing to at least a queen-size mattress to provide both of you enough room to stretch out. Just remember one thing — you'll have to match a mattress's firmness to suit both your needs.

Take a test run. "The most important thing when shopping for a mattress is to take the time to try it out in the store," Butler says. "Spend a good five minutes testing it out." You might be a little embarrassed at first, but don't let that hold you back. "Lie down on your back and then get into your usual sleep position," she says. "Be willing to stretch."

Take notice of how the bed supports your pressure points, like your hips and your shoulders. It should conform to your body, not cut off your circulation. And firmness is not all that it's cracked up to be. "The mattress doesn't have to be hard as a board," Butler states. "The word is support, not firmness. You can get firmness and still get cushy layers on top."

Learn the basics. Because of the wonders of modern technology, you have almost as many types of mattresses to choose from as there are feathers in your pillow. Here are the major types:

- **Innerspring coils.** The American Chiropractic Association recommends this type. Each coil can adjust differently to your body, so it can mold itself perfectly to the natural curve of your spine.

- **Airbeds.** In a small study of back pain sufferers, air mattresses eased the pain of 95 percent of the participants. About 88 percent of them slept better than they did on their mattresses at home. An airbed's firmness is adjustable, which might explain why they work so well. With some of the models, you can even set each side of the mattress to a different firmness setting.

- **Latex.** Experts specially design these mattresses to match your height and weight. You can also choose different firmness settings on each side.

- **Waterbeds.** The ripples and waves aren't for everyone, and experts still disagree whether they provide enough support for your back. But if you like the way a waterbed feels, go for it.

When considering all of the different varieties of mattresses, Butler compares them to athletic shoes. There are so many brands, each constructed in different ways with different materials, but one isn't necessarily better than another. "What feels comfortable to you," that's what counts, according to Butler.

Price it right. When you're considering mattresses, Butler suggests, remember the old saying, "You get what you pay for." Just think, you spend about one-third of your life in bed. Don't settle for a poor-quality mattress just to save a few dollars. For waterbeds, that's doubly true. A well-crafted waterbed could save you from an unexpected late-night swim.

Shop around. You can still nab a great deal while buying your dream mattress. That is, if you check all of your shopping options. Today, there are a lot of them — mattress superstores, online shops, mail-order warehouses. Look for stores that have the best perks, like free delivery, comfort guarantees, and flexibility on prices.

OSTEOARTHRITIS

Sidestep injury to avoid OA

What do Dorothy Hamill, Jimmy Connors, and Hank Aaron have in common? Besides being former world-class athletes, they all have osteoarthritis (OA). Experts think the disease may stem from injuries they suffered in pursuing their athletic dreams. So if you have a sports injury, you too may be at risk for this type of arthritis.

Evidence supporting a link between joint injuries and later development of OA comes from a study of more than 1,000 graduates of Johns Hopkins Medical School. Those who injured their joints as young adults were more than twice as likely to have OA in their later years, researchers found. The odds were even worse for specific injuries. People with hip problems were three times more likely to get OA of the hip, and knee injuries made a person five times more likely to develop OA of the knee.

> ### What is it?
>
> The "wear and tear" of life plays a big part in developing this disease. Over time, the cushiony tissue in your joints, called cartilage, wears down. Without it, the ends of your bones rub together, causing pain and difficulty moving. Osteoarthritis can occur in any joint, but especially in your hands, hips, back, and knees.
>
> Symptoms:
> - Steady or occasional joint pain
> - Morning stiffness
> - Swollen or tender joints
> - Cracking sound or feeling in a joint

If you want to put the odds in your favor, you need to protect your joints from injury. Follow these preventive steps so you can enjoy your golden years without falling victim to this crippling disease.

Play smart. Unless you plan to play for the NFL, avoid sports like football that put heavy stress on your joints. Even if your days of playing team sports are just a memory, you need to be careful. Pitching baseballs to your grandson can be rough on your shoulder if you're not throwing the ball just right. And if you decide to take up tennis or golf, be sure to get proper instruction on technique from a pro. Without guidance, you can injure yourself just as easily in a non-contact sport.

Get equipped. No matter which sport you choose to keep in shape, be sure to use the proper equipment. Runners need good, shock-absorbing running shoes, and tennis players need shoes designed specifically for stop-and-go movements. Scientists spend years and millions of research dollars designing equipment that can protect you from injury. So take advantage of technology.

Stay fit. Build up the muscles in front of your thighs, experts say, and you decrease the chance of injuring your knees. Studies show that increasing the strength of these muscles by 25 percent can cut your risk of OA by roughly the same percentage.

Try a combination of aerobic exercises like walking or swimming, strength training, and range-of-motion exercises to help keep joints limber. Make it a point to exercise every day so you don't end up like the "weekend warriors" seen in emergency rooms every Saturday and Sunday.

Stay light. Extra weight puts added stress on your joints, especially your knees. That additional weight can cause your cartilage to start wearing away, giving OA an opening. Researchers found that people who lost as little as 11 pounds were able to cut their arthritis risk in half. In the circle of fitness, staying light makes it easier to exercise, which in turn, helps keep you light.

Get treatment. If you do hurt yourself, don't hobble around or make a homemade sling. Pain is your body's way of telling you something is wrong. Let your doctor decide what treatment is right for you. He or she may want to immobilize a bone or joint so it can heal better and lessen your risk of arthritis. You might have to wear a brace to avoid further damage.

Get rest. Don't let your enthusiasm for a sport be your downfall. Rest is an important part of the healing process, and it can make you stronger in the long run. You can permanently damage your joints and increase your chances of getting OA if you keep playing despite an injury. Doctors are now able to completely replace knees and hips if necessary, but in the meantime, take good care of the ones you have.

3 natural ways to repair your joints

Did you hear the one about the doctors who turned fat into cartilage? No, it's not a joke or the plot of a science fiction thriller. Believe it or not, scientists at Duke University are working on a procedure that would allow you to use your own fat to rebuild your arthritic joints. In a few years, it could be reality. The researchers have already succeeded in "training" fat cells in a test tube to become cartilage, the connective tissue that lines your joints. Eventually, they hope to inject this miraculous substance into injured or arthritic joints to help your body heal itself naturally.

If your joints are in need of repair, though, don't wait for this amazing procedure. Rebuild your joints now — naturally — and relieve the pain of your arthritis today.

Douse your joints with vitamin D. This nutrient should be high on your list of arthritis-fighters because it protects the cartilage and bones in your joints. And it's easy to get, too. Just spend some time each day out in the sunshine. Amazingly, your skin can turn five minutes of sunlight, two or three days a week, into all the vitamin D you need. If you have dark skin or live in a colder climate, you might need more sunlight, so increase your vitamin D by eating fortified dairy foods, seafood, and eggs.

Although it's important to get your daily requirement of vitamin D, taking more may help if you have osteoarthritis of the knee. An eight-year study found that taking higher doses of vitamin D than normally recommended helped control knee pain. Don't take a supplement without checking with your doctor, though, because too much can be toxic.

Care for your cartilage with vitamin C. Without this critical vitamin, your body could not make collagen, the all-important building block for cartilage, muscles, tendons, and bone. This means you risk damaging your joints if you don't get enough vitamin C. Experts say your joints can weaken three times faster without this nutrient than if you take in enough.

Vitamin C is also important because it's an antioxidant that naturally fights damage in many parts of your body. A study at Boston University's Medical Center found that knee cartilage is one of the areas it helps. In the study, people who ate foods high in vitamin C had less pain and found their disease progressed more slowly than those who ate less vitamin C. So enjoy plenty of oranges, strawberries, and red peppers, and see if your joints feel a little better.

Wash away arthritis troubles with water. Making new cartilage for your joints could be as simple as drinking eight 8-ounce glasses of water each day. This crystal-clear beverage is a key ingredient in that joint-protecting tissue. Water also forms a cushion that helps lubricate your joints, which makes them easier to bend and move around.

Paying attention to your nutritional needs may be just a small part of your arthritis treatment, but it's an important one. It won't cure your osteoarthritis or keep it from getting worse, but it may help improve your quality of life. And who knows? Maybe someday a cure will be as easy as going in for a "tummy tuck" and coming out with a newly rebuilt knee.

Don't get burned by topical creams

Ahhh. That pain-relieving ointment feels like an aspirin on your achy spots.

Well, that's because it is, basically. Many topical rubs use salicylates, the main ingredient in aspirin, to help relieve the pain. But if you're allergic to aspirin, this could mean trouble. You could have a reaction when the medicine is absorbed by your body.

If you experience ringing in your ears, blurred vision, or shortness of breath, stop using the cream immediately and tell your doctor about it.

Salicylates also may interact with certain drugs, such as warfarin, so watch for symptoms if you take prescription medications. If you know you are allergic to aspirin, read labels carefully and avoid any product containing salicylates.

Vanquish OA with vegetables

Your mother told you that eating your vegetables would keep you healthy, and she was right. Now scientists say certain vegetables might even protect you from osteoarthritis (OA).

Researchers at the University of North Carolina at Chapel Hill found that vitamin E and other antioxidants in brightly colored vegetables seem to protect your knees from OA. Blood samples taken from healthy people as well as people with OA told the story of who was listening to mom's advice and who wasn't.

The researchers measured the levels of 11 antioxidant phytochemicals in each of 400 subjects of different races. "We found vitamin E, also called alpha tocopherol, to be associated with about 30 percent lower risk of knee osteoarthritis in whites," says assistant research professor Dr. Joanne Jordan. "We did not see a protective effect in blacks but don't know why."

Other antioxidants — beta cryptoxanthine, lutein, and lycopene — appeared to lower the chances of getting OA of the knee by 30 to 40 percent, Jordan says. These phytochemicals, which are common in orange and green vegetables and tomatoes, put you ahead of the game when it comes to arthritis protection.

Fight OA with E. Vitamin E is available in most raw oils, but heating it to high temperatures destroys it. So if your diet consists mainly of fried or highly processed foods, you're not getting the benefit of this antioxidant. Also, if you've been on a low-fat diet for a long time, you could be low in vitamin E. Make an effort to get more of this valuable vitamin into your diet. Good sources include plant foods, especially wheat germ, soybeans, sunflower seeds, and almonds.

Pick the bright ones. Like the captain of the debate team choosing his speakers, you should pick the bright ones. As Jordan's study showed, colorful vegetables are full of the antioxidants that protect you from inflammatory diseases like arthritis.

Take your pick of yellow-orange fruits and vegetables such as apricots, cantaloupe, carrots, mangoes, papaya, peaches, sweet potatoes, pumpkin, and winter squash. In addition, eat plenty of dark green veggies such as broccoli, collard greens, and spinach. Try a couple from each color group daily to get a variety of vitamins and antioxidants in your diet. One caution about tomatoes, though. They're a good source of lycopene, but some experts think they might aggravate OA if you already have the disease.

Spice up your plate. If you want even more protection for your joints, sprinkle your veggies with spices. Ginger and turmeric are good choices — they have a phytochemical called curcumin that helps reduce inflammation. Studies show it can work as well as non-steroidal anti-inflammatory drugs (NSAIDs) without the side effects.

Look for these spices at the grocery store, and use them to perk up a stir-fry or vegetable dish. Or try ginger tea for a spicy antioxidant pick-me-up. But be careful if you take NSAIDs or blood-thinning medicines like warfarin. These spices can add to the effect of those drugs, so talk to your doctor before using them.

Recharge your joints with glucosamine

There's good news for you if you are among the growing number of people considering glucosamine sulfate for relief from the pain of osteoarthritis (OA).

Glucosamine, found naturally in the body, gives strength and rigidity to the cartilage that cushions your joints and keeps your bones from rubbing together. Glucosamine supplements are supposed to help rebuild your damaged cartilage, but most research has not been clear on the benefits of glucosamine in treating osteoarthritis.

A new long-term study from Belgium, however, presents convincing evidence glucosamine can bring long-lasting pain relief to your aching knees. In the study, those with OA who took 1,500 milligrams (mg) of glucosamine daily reported less pain and disability. And those good results continued throughout the full three years of the study.

Researchers also found evidence that glucosamine helps prevent wearing away of cartilage in the knees. Those who took placebos, pills that contained no active ingredients, lost space between the bones of their joints during the study. But those taking glucosamine had no significant narrowing of joint space.

You'll need patience if you decide to take glucosamine since it takes about a month to get results and perhaps eight to 12 weeks for the full effect. Nonsteroidal anti-inflammatory drugs (NSAIDs), such as aspirin, acetaminophen, and ibuprofen, act faster on OA pain, but they can cause gastrointestinal bleeding and liver damage. Glucosamine, on the other hand, doesn't seem to have any serious side effects. And once it kicks in, it's likely to be just as effective as the NSAIDs.

You can buy glucosamine by itself or combined with another supplement, chondroitin, which is also effective in relieving knee pain and improving mobility. Chondroitin is available by itself, too, and appears to have even fewer side effects then glucosamine. But both are made from animal products — glucosamine from clamshells and chondroitin from cow tracheas — so be aware of possible allergic reactions.

Whether you consider taking glucosamine, chondroitin, or the combined supplements, the Arthritis Foundation offers these suggestions:

- ✤ Don't stop taking your current medications without talking to your doctor. Discuss the potential benefits and any possible allergic reactions or other problems that might arise from taking these supplements alone or in combination with your other medicines.

- ✤ Be sure you actually have OA. These supplements are not recommended for other kinds of arthritis. If you have joint pain and you think it might be caused by OA, see a doctor, preferably a rheumatologist, for an accurate diagnosis.

- ✤ Children and pregnant women should not take glucosamine or chondroitin supplements since the safety and side effects aren't yet clear for these groups.

- ✤ If you have diabetes, consult your doctor about glucosamine. It's an amino sugar, so you may need to have your blood sugar levels tested more often if you take it.

- ✤ Be careful about taking chondroitin if you're on blood thinners, including aspirin. It has a similar molecular makeup to the blood-thinner heparin.

The FDA does not regulate dietary supplements, so be sure to buy them from well-known companies. Read the labels carefully, and look for those that give you a total of 1,500 mg of glucosamine. The usual dosage is 500 mg three times a day. For chondroitin, aim for 1,200 mg total, or 400 mg three times a day. Again, discuss these supplements with your doctor first, so she can help decide if they're an appropriate treatment for your arthritis.

Get the scoop on supplements

Confusion over which brand is best could leave you with aching knees long after you begin taking glucosamine and chondroitin. With so many choices and no government regulation, how do you know what to pick? One way is to look for the ConsumerLabs.com flask-shaped seal of approval on the container.

ConsumerLabs regularly tests supplements to see if their labels accurately reflect their contents. In looking at 25 brands of glucosamine, chondroitin, and a combination of the two, ConsumerLabs found the glucosamine samples fared the best. All of them contained the amounts listed on their labels. But neither of the two chondroitin supplements passed, and only half the combined supplements had the amounts of chondroitin listed.

ConsumerLabs also checked the supplements for manganese, a nutrient that helps your bones. More than 11 mg daily can cause problems with your nervous system. Some supplements contained as much as 25 mg to 30 mg of manganese in the recommended daily dosage. It's easy to get all the manganese you need from tea, nuts, beans, and whole grains, so read labels and avoid it in supplements.

To see the studies and a list of ConsumerLabs' approved supplements, you can subscribe to ConsumerLabs.com at <www.consumerlabs.com>.

Women: Reduce your risk of OA

Being a woman has its advantages. Osteoarthritis is not one of them. According to the Arthritis Foundation, 15.3 million women have this painful condition, making up about three-fourths of all osteoarthritis (OA) cases. The risks become even worse as you get older — women over 65 are more than twice as likely to develop osteoarthritis of the knee as men the same age.

Why women are more at risk is something of a mystery. It could be a result of weaker cartilage and tendons. Or it could have something to do with decreasing levels of estrogen after menopause. Whatever the reason, if you're a woman, you need to be especially careful.

Shed some weight. Heavy women carry a heavier risk. Every pound you put on means 2 to 3 pounds of extra pressure on your knees. But in one study, overweight women who lost an average of 11 pounds slashed their risk for osteoarthritis of the knees in half. It's best to lose weight gradually, however, combining a proper diet with more exercise.

Build up your legs. Weak quadriceps, or thigh muscles, can contribute to osteoarthritis of the knee. Increasing your leg strength by just 25 percent could decrease your risk of OA by 20 to 30 percent. Even if you already have osteoarthritis, exercising for strength and endurance is important. Ask an expert to help you design a low-intensity workout that helps you stay mobile and flexible without causing pain.

Go shoe shopping. High heels spell trouble. And not just those ultra-stylish — and uncomfortable — stiletto heels. Wide heels actually cause more twisting force on your knees, putting you at greater risk for osteoarthritis. Because they're more comfortable than skinnier heels, you're more likely to wear them longer — and do more damage.

Your best bet is to avoid high heels altogether. If you already have osteoarthritis, look for shock-absorbing footwear or try putting heel wedges in your shoes to cushion the stress on your knees.

Consider HRT. The jury is still out on this one, but because osteoarthritis strikes so many women after menopause, many believe it's linked to an estrogen deficiency. Some research shows that postmenopausal women who take estrogen for at least five years have more knee cartilage than women who don't. More cartilage means more protection against osteoarthritis.

However, other studies show estrogen has no effect — or even increases your risk of OA. Discuss the pros and cons of hormone replacement therapy (HRT) with your doctor.

Check out surgery. The facts are more women than men suffer from OA of the hip or knee. And women typically experience more pain and require more assistance for day-to-day tasks because of it.

In spite of this, according to a recent study in *The New England Journal of Medicine*, women are much less likely to have joint replacement surgery than men.

Don't be afraid to ask your doctor or an orthopedic surgeon about this highly safe and effective option. It might be your best weapon against osteoarthritis.

The lowdown on NSAIDs

Acetaminophen (Tylenol) is usually the drug of choice for osteoarthritis since it can relieve pain with few side effects. If you need something stronger, your doctor likely will prescribe non-steroidal anti-inflammatory drugs (NSAIDs). Although these drugs can be effective, long-term use also carries some risk. Check the following chart to see what you should look for.

Type of Drug	Used for	Warning
Acetylsalicylic acid **Generic name:** aspirin **Brand names:** Anacin, Bayer, Bufferin, Easprin, Zorprin	Inexpensive pain relief	Possible stomach irritation (buy enteric-coated pills to protect stomach); lessens blood clotting ability, which could lead to increased bleeding
Nonacetylated salicylates **Generic names:** choline magnesium trisalicylate, salsalate **Brand names:** Trilisate, Disalcid	People at risk for ulcers and GI bleeding, or those with damaged kidneys	Not always effective for pain relief compared to other NSAIDs
COX-2 inhibitors **Generic names:** celecoxib, rofecoxib **Brand names:** Celebrex, Vioxx	Arthritis symptoms specifically	Can still irritate GI tract and cause ulcers, although to a lesser degree than other NSAIDs
Enolic acid **Generic name:** meloxicam **Brand name:** Mobic	Pain and stiffness of osteoarthritis	Rarely, can cause GI bleeding
Fenamate **Generic name:** Meclofenamate	Osteoarthritis of spine and peripheral joints	Can cause bowel irritation that occasionally leads to bowel disease

Type of Drug	Used for	Warning
Keto-napthylalkanone **Generic name:** nabumetone **Brand name:** Relafen	Pain relief	No specific warning
Phenylbutazone **Generic name:** phenylbutazone	Strong, short-term relief for severe osteoarthritis pain	May lead to bone marrow toxicity
Indole-Indene acetic acid derivatives **Generic names:** diclofenac, diclofenac/misoprostol, etodolac, indomethacin, sulindac, tolmetin **Brand names:** Voltaren, Arthrotec, Lodine, Indocin, Clinoril, Tolectin	Severe arthritis	Can cause central nervous system side effects such as convulsions or forgetfulness
Propionic acid derivatives **Generic names:** fenoprofen calcium, ibuprofen, ketoprofen, naproxen **Brand names:** Nalfon, Advil, Motrin, Actron, Orudis, Naprosyn, Anaprox, Aleve	Pain relief	Fenoprofen must not be taken with food

OSTEOPOROSIS

Warning: Eating fat can thin your bones

That piece of pie or bowl of chips will not only lead to an overweight body and an overworked heart, but to thin, fragile bones, as well.

It's a new concept but one experts say makes sense. A high-fat diet means high cholesterol. And high cholesterol is now associated with fewer bone-forming cells in your body. Traditional remedies for osteoporosis target only the cells that break down bone. But it's just as important you protect the cells that build up your bones. That means cutting the fat out of your menu and lowering your cholesterol.

You can do this by eating lean meats, low-fat dairy products, and healthy carbohydrates. Here are some additional tips for cutting the fat but not the flavor.

Feast on fiber. Filling up on fiber-rich foods is an excellent way to lower cholesterol. Soluble fiber — the kind that dissolves easily in water — slows down your food as it passes through your stomach and small intestine. This means your body has more time to pull out the bad cholesterol and get rid of it.

The American Heart Association recommends lowering your cholesterol with oatmeal, oat bran, rice bran, beans, barley, citrus fruits, strawberries, and apples. A bowl of high-fiber cereal in the morning is a great way to start the day and save your bones.

Change your oil. Monounsaturated fat, the kind in olive oil, cuts down on your bad cholesterol without harming the good. Instead of cooking with other vegetable oils or butter, sauté your food in olive oil, wine, or broth. Add herbs and spices for more flavor.

Bake without butter. When a baking recipe calls for butter or oil, fat-watchers often use applesauce or puréed prunes instead. A recent study found another surprising fat substitute — pawpaw purée.

The pawpaw is an oblong, yellow-green fruit that grows in the eastern U.S. and Canada, and tastes a little like a mango or banana. If you mash the pulp in a blender or food processor, you end up with a healthy alternative to oil.

People ate muffins made with vegetable oil, applesauce, or pawpaws. They thought the pawpaw muffins were as tasty as the full-fat muffins. If pawpaw purée sounds appealing to you, maybe banana or pumpkin would be other fat-free alternatives you'd like to try.

> ### *What is it?*
>
> Osteoporosis (meaning "porous bones") is a disease where your bones slowly lose density, making them fragile and more likely to break. It usually occurs because you have low levels of calcium and other minerals important to bone health. Your spinal column, wrists, and hips are the most common fracture sites, and even mild stress can cause an injury.
>
> Symptoms:
> - Stooping posture ("widow's hump")
> - Gradual decrease in height
> - Back pain
> - Broken bones

Double your defense against double danger

If you've got thinning bones, you may have heart disease, too. At least in women, low bone density appears to go hand in hand with hardening of the arteries. So, if you're fighting one disease, you might as well fight them both. Follow these proven steps to a healthier heart and beefier bones.

Cash in on calcium-rich foods. If you're over 50, you need 1,200 milligrams (mg) of calcium every day. Of course, dairy foods are the top sources of this bone-building mineral, but you'd be surprised what other foods can deliver calcium to your plate.

Food	Serving Size	Calcium (mg)
Skim milk	8 ounces	302
Low-fat, fruit yogurt	8 ounces	300
Swiss cheese	1 ounce	272
Dried figs	10 figs	269
Tofu, firm	1/2 cup	258
Mozzarella cheese	1 ounce	183
Collards, boiled	1/2 cup	179
Blackstrap molasses	1 tablespoon	172
Cottage cheese	1 cup	126
Sardines, in oil	2 sardines	92
Mustard greens, boiled	1/2 cup	52
Kale, boiled	1/2 cup	47
Broccoli, boiled	1/2 cup	36

Look for other non-dairy foods fortified with calcium, like breakfast cereals and orange juice.

By increasing your calcium intake, you'll not only get a nutrient vital to healthy blood pressure and cholesterol levels, but also a steady heartbeat.

Pounce on produce. The more fruits and veggies you eat, the stronger your bones. At least that's what some research says. A group of men increased bone density and lowered their risk of breaking a hip with every extra vegetable or fruit serving they ate per day. There's a good chance that magnesium and potassium are behind these amazing results. Your body needs those two essential minerals to take advantage of calcium and build bones.

For a healthy heart, it's also important to make potassium and magnesium key ingredients in your daily diet. They are essential for keeping your arteries clear, your heart strong, and your cholesterol and blood pressure low.

Avocados, prunes, and dried figs and apricots provide potent potassium stores. For marvelous amounts of magnesium, munch on nuts, beans, cereals, bananas, and oranges.

Shake off your taste for salt. In your body, calcium and salt compete in a race to get absorbed. Sometimes extra salt wins and calcium passes right on out. In addition, when you eat too much salt, your kidneys work especially hard to flush it out — and they often end up flushing out other important minerals, like calcium, too.

Need another reason to slow down on salt? The connection between a high-salt diet and high blood pressure is well known. Even if salt doesn't affect everyone this way, play it safe for the sake of your heart and bones.

Fight back with estrogen. Start taking estrogen early and you could cut your risk of hip fracture in half. No wonder hormone replacement therapy (HRT) is the most common prescription to fight osteoporosis.

Estrogen plays a direct role in how well your body builds bone, and it may help with calcium absorption. To get the most benefit from HRT, experts recommend beginning a program as soon as you notice the first signs of menopause. If you've been menopausal for years now, don't worry — HRT still seems to be beneficial. It's shown to increase hip and spine bone mass by 5 to 10 percent.

You'll also help your heart since estrogen appears to lower your cholesterol, keep your blood flowing smoothly, and reduce your chances of stroke.

Remember, though, HRT can have troubling side effects — including an increased risk of breast cancer. Meet with your doctor and weigh the upside and the downside before starting HRT.

Lose weight without losing bone. Here's the skinny on weight loss — dropping too many pounds could actually lower your bone mass and put you at risk for osteoporosis. Some think a lower body weight puts less stress on your bones, slowing down the rate they make new cells. Or less weight could mean less fat, cutting down on the amount of estrogen that's available.

Either way, this doesn't give you the green light to put on the pounds. Instead, live at a sensible, healthy weight. Talk to your doctor about what weight matches your body frame, sex, and age. Then, achieve it with a balanced diet and exercise. Working out, don't forget, builds up bones while burning calories. And experts believe an amazing 50 to 70 percent of all heart disease cases stem from obesity. That's enough to make your heart flutter.

Boost your bones with exercise

Now is the time to take that dancing class you've been dreaming about. It could improve the thickness of your bones by up to 10 percent. Or hit the gym, and add an amazing 30 percent to your bone mass.

Exercise cannot only build up your bones, it can also pump up your muscles. With stronger muscles, you'll have better balance, an easier time getting around, more independence, and an overall healthier life.

So, if you want to halt the advance of osteoporosis and take charge of feeling good, start a daily exercise routine.

Stand on your own two feet. Dedication to exercise can protect you from bone loss throughout your life. And weight-bearing exercises are the first step.

These include any activity that works against gravity, forcing you to carry the weight of your body on your feet, legs, and hips. You can walk, jog, or engage in more demanding activities like playing soccer or dancing.

Participate in weight-bearing exercises at least three or four times a week. Just like muscles, bones get stronger the more you use them.

Resist weak bones. If you want to keep your bones thick and strong, you'll need resistance training, too. These exercises use your muscles to lift, push, or pull weights. You can try dumbbells, barbells, or the weight machines at your local fitness center.

Isometric exercises are a type of resistance training — you tighten your muscles but don't move your joints. They are excellent if you're a beginner or if you suffer from arthritis. You can do them in the comfort of your own home, but they'll have you strutting your stuff around a gym in no time. Here are two you can try.

- ↜ Hold your hands in front of your abdomen with your palms together as if you're about to clap. Push your elbows away from your body, and press your palms together for five seconds. Don't hold your breath.

- ↜ Sit on the edge of a chair with your legs stretched straight out in front of you. With your heels resting on the ground, point your toes towards the ceiling. You should feel your shin muscle tighten. Straighten your knee, pushing it down until you feel the muscles on the back of your thigh stretch.

To pump your muscles up some more, add these joint-bending, or isotonic, exercises to your program.

↫ Sit in a chair with your knees bent and your feet on the ground. Straighten one of your legs and lift it off the ground until you feel the muscles on the front of your leg tense. Lower it back to the ground and repeat with the other leg.

↫ Stand in front of a wall. Place both your hands flat on the wall at shoulder height and shuffle your feet backward slightly. You should feel the weight in your shoulders and chest. Bend your elbows and drop halfway to the wall. Then push back, straightening your elbows.

Do these exercises gently at first and just a few times each. Gauge your body's reaction and gradually increase the repetitions. You'll be surprised by your progress.

Make the sky your limit. You need to keep pushing yourself if you want to reach new heights of bone and muscle strength. In other words, you must branch out with more difficult exercises to keep getting the same bone-building effect. Weights and resistance machines are perfect for this, since you can always add heavier weights.

To set up a tougher workout routine, ask your doctor to recommend a physical trainer. Or just stop by your local gym or YMCA. These places usually have a staff of physical trainers who can give advice and sometimes even a free training session.

Remember, though, don't work yourself too long or too hard, especially when you're just beginning. Pay attention to your body for signs you should stop. And always warm up, breathe, don't rush, and cool down.

Don't give up. You can never stop exercising. Once you drop your workout routine, all of the progress you made will disappear quicker than it takes to say "sweatband." In one recent study, women lost 12 month's of hard-earned bone mass after they stopped exercising for just six months.

If you think you have an excuse because you're "too old," think again. Even the most frail seniors appear to benefit from resistance training. If you're wheelchair-bound, you can still improve your strength and become more independent. Exercise may also help you heal quicker. According to research, if you're active you could spend less time in the hospital than your peers who don't exercise.

Check with your doctor. Whatever form of exercise you choose, talk with your doctor first, especially if you suffer from chronic conditions like heart disease.

Get the story on supplements

Picking the right calcium supplement — carbonate or citrate — can be tricky business. Don't give up though, because, chances are, you're falling short of the recommended daily intake of 1,200 milligrams (mg).

Of course, according to experts, the best way to get bone-building calcium is to squeeze as many calcium-rich foods into your daily diet as you can. However, if you still have trouble reaching your goal, then turn to supplements.

Consider the side effects. Most agree — calcium carbonate can cause side effects. You'll mainly experience minor tummy problems, like constipation, bloating, and gas. To straighten out the trouble, try drinking more water. If you can't live with the discomfort, switch to calcium citrate.

Compare labels. Not all supplements are created equal. Some contain more "elemental," or actual, calcium than others. You'll find anywhere from 150 to 600 mg in one tablet.

That means you must read the label for the elemental calcium per dose. Then, you'll have to do a little math to figure out exactly how many doses you'll need to meet your daily requirement. For instance, you'd need two tablets of a product containing 600 mg of elemental calcium per tablet. But you'd need four of another product containing 300 mg per tablet.

Having to take only one calcium carbonate pill compared to five calcium citrate pills could be a big deal.

Assure absorption. Whatever supplement you choose, it won't do you any good if your body can't use it. According to Dr. Robert P. Heaney, a member of the board of directors of the National Osteoporosis Foundation, the U.S. Food and Drug Administration does not test to see how well calcium gets absorbed in the body.

He suggests choosing a brand name supplement whose manufacturer may be more aware of purity levels. And go with chewables. You naturally break these supplements up and make them more absorbable.

Look out for lead. Your calcium supplement might also be giving you more than just calcium. A recent study in the *Journal of the American Medical Association* reported that some over-the-counter calcium carbonate brands contain lead, a natural but very toxic metal that gets mixed in with calcium during mining. Even name brand calcium supplements labeled "natural" or "refined" contain some amount of lead.

If you're like most people and simply supplement with calcium, don't worry too much about these findings. None of the brands tested contained more than the daily recommended limit of lead (6 micrograms). That makes your risk of lead poisoning far less likely than your risk of not getting enough calcium. So, don't stop taking those supplements.

Nevertheless, according to the researchers, any level of lead is a bad level of lead. They suggest only buying calcium supplements that say "essentially lead free" on the label. It's especially important if you:

- ❧ have a kidney condition that requires extra calcium.
- ❧ take megadoses of vitamin and mineral supplements.
- ❧ are lactose intolerant and get all your calcium from supplements.

Track your intake. Too much calcium can be as bad as too little. Unless your doctor says otherwise, don't take 1,200 mg — your entire recommended daily amount — in supplements. Instead, roughly estimate how much calcium you get from food and subtract that from 1,200 mg. Then make up the difference with supplements.

If you push your daily calcium intake as high as 2,500 mg, you could put yourself at risk for deficiencies in iron and zinc. Calcium can interfere with your body's use of these nutrients, as well as with medications like bisphosphonates and tetracycline.

Too much calcium can also mean kidney problems. In fact, if you're prone to kidney stones, talk with your doctor before taking any kind of calcium supplement.

Eat at the proper time. If you want your body to totally absorb your supplement, you must take it at specific times. Take calcium carbonate with meals, and calcium citrate on an empty stomach.

Double up with D. Getting more vitamin D means your body can absorb and use calcium better. If you're over 70, be even more careful to get the recommended amount of D — 15 micrograms a day. As you age, your skin doesn't produce as much of this vitamin from sunlight, and your digestive track doesn't absorb it as well as it used to. Talk with your doctor about vitamin D supplements.

Be certain of soy's calcium

You could be getting a lot less calcium than you suspect. This warning comes from Dr. Robert P. Heaney of the Osteoporosis Research Center at Creighton University.

He means your body can't absorb the calcium from fortified soy milk as easily as it does from cow's milk. In fact, you absorb about 75 percent less. The problem lies within certain chemicals in the soy milk called antiabsorbers. These seem to limit how well your body takes in and uses the calcium.

This problem isn't going away anytime soon since the FDA regulates calcium as a food and not as a drug. That means the government measures how much calcium is in a product, but not how much your body will absorb.

Heaney has three recommendations if you're concerned about getting enough calcium from soy milk.

Look on the labels. In its natural state, soy milk contains low levels of calcium — only about 10 milligrams (mg) in every cup. And remember, your body absorbs only a small percentage of that. On the other hand, a cup of cow's milk contains over 350 mg of calcium and you can use most of it. So, soy milk producers fortify their products with extra calcium to make them more attractive to consumers. These products can contain anywhere from 80 to 500 mg of calcium per cup.

It's important then, Heaney says, to buy the brand that gives you the most calcium bang for your buck. "Go with brand names. They have their reputations on the line."

Supersize your servings. "Drink a third to a half more of soy milk," Heaney advises. This should give your body the actual calcium amount on the label. For instance, instead of drinking a 12-ounce serving, pour yourself a tall glass of 16 to 18 ounces.

Shop for other sources. "Seek out other calcium-fortified foods and drinks," Heaney says. Fortified orange juice and breakfast cereals are two top choices. Natural non-dairy sources, like legumes, leafy greens, and broccoli, are always a healthy idea, too.

Getting enough calcium from your diet is only one part of operation osteoporosis prevention. To keep your bones strong and healthy, Heaney says it's important to exercise, keep a sensible body weight, quit smoking, take in enough vitamin D, and, if you're a woman, keep your hormones in balance.

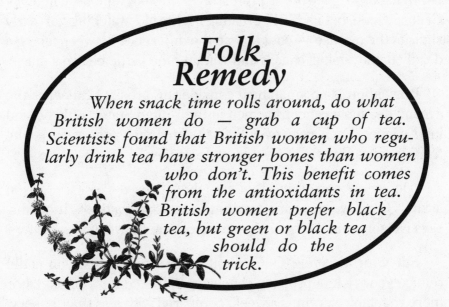

Folk Remedy

When snack time rolls around, do what British women do — grab a cup of tea. Scientists found that British women who regularly drink tea have stronger bones than women who don't. This benefit comes from the antioxidants in tea. British women prefer black tea, but green or black tea should do the trick.

PROSTATE CANCER

Proven protection against prostate cancer

Lifestyle is probably the major cause of prostate cancer, says Dr. William G. Nelson, a professor at Johns Hopkins Oncology Center. Good habits — like eating right and watching for early signs of the disease — could mean the difference between facing a deadly battle against cancer and winning the battle before it starts.

Prevention is no small deal considering prostate cancer is the second deadliest cancer for men in the United States, only behind lung cancer. Each year over 200,000 American men receive the terrible news that they have prostate cancer.

"Do we eat something that somehow causes cancer?" Nelson asks. "Or do we not eat something that's protective?" It seems, says Nelson, that the truth is somewhere in between.

Eat your veggies. One recent study showed that you could reduce your risk of prostate cancer by 35 percent if you eat 24 or more vegetable servings a week, compared with less than 14 servings. Unfortunately, not all vegetables are created equal. The brassica, or cruciferous, family of vegetables stood out in this study. These include broccoli, cauliflower, brussels sprouts, kohlrabi, and cabbage. Study participants who ate these vegetables three or more times a week lowered their prostate cancer risk by over 40 percent. They all contain sulfurophanes, chemicals that neutralize cancer-causing substances before they can do any damage.

Serve healthy fats. "The less red meat idea," Nelson adds, "is not a bad idea." Recently, one study reported that men who eat five or more servings of red meat every week could be increasing their risk of prostate cancer by almost 80 percent.

If you eat fish instead of red meat, you'll be cutting back on harmful saturated fat. You'll also be getting omega-3 fatty acids, "good" fats that seem to protect against cancer. Men who frequently eat fish are up to three times less likely to get prostate cancer than men who eat little or no fish. Fatty fish rich in omega-3 fatty acids, like salmon, herring, and mackerel, seem to take the biggest bite out of cancer.

Monounsaturated fatty acids (MUFAs) are also another beneficial kind of fat. Experts have known they're good for your heart, but now they believe MUFAs also protect your prostate. In one recent study, subjects who ate at least one teaspoon of olive, canola, or peanut oil a day — all good sources of MUFAs — had a 50-percent lower risk of cancer than the people who didn't get MUFAs in their diet. Eating peanuts and avocados is another great way to punch up your MUFA intake.

> ### *What is it?*
>
> Your prostate is a gland that makes and stores semen. It is located below your bladder and surrounds the tube that carries urine out of your body. When cells in your prostate become cancerous, they divide and grow until they form a mass of tissue called a tumor. This tumor can press against your urethra and bladder.
>
> Symptoms:
> - Frequent or difficult urination
> - Dribbling
> - Blood in urine
> - Painful urination
> - Painful ejaculation
> - Hip or back pain

Fight back with flaxseed. According to a new study from Duke University, flaxseed kills cancer cells in their tracks. You can thank flaxseed's high levels of omega-3 fatty acids, fiber, and lignan.

Adding these tiny seeds to your diet is easy. Sprinkle them on cereal and yogurt, and throw some into your batter or dough when you're baking. For maximum benefits, grind them first. Look for flaxseed at your local health food store or supermarket. You can also buy flaxseed oil. It's an excellent substitute for your usual salad dressing oil, but don't cook with it. Flaxseed oil can actually break down into harmful compounds when it's heated.

Guard yourself with green tea. Green tea could be one reason why men in Asia have far fewer cases of prostate cancer than Western men. Experts believe chemicals in the tea called catechins act like sharpshooters, tracking down tumor cells before they can harm healthy prostate cells. If you'd like to cash in on this ancient Asian secret, buy bags or loose leaves of green tea at your local grocery or health food store. Steep the tea in hot, but not boiling, water for about three minutes and sip it before it cools.

Take charge with these nutrients. Experts also point to specific nutrients that could have extra strong protective powers.

- **Quercetin.** This natural flavonoid seems to stop tumor cells from growing. It's found in foods from apples, onions, and leafy greens to red wine and tea.

- **Beta carotene.** Even though it's from the Dead Sea, an alga called *Dunaliella bardawil* could give new life to your prostate. That's because it's loaded with beta carotene. A recent study found that men with low levels of beta carotene were 45 percent more likely to develop prostate cancer than men with high levels. Because of its antioxidant abilities, beta carotene could boost your immune system and protect your heart, too. Besides *Dunaliella*, look for beta carotene in carrots, spinach, sweet potatoes, and apricots.

- **Selenium.** "It looks like selenium supplements reduced the number of prostate cancers diagnosed," Nelson says about a recent study. Getting the recommended dietary allowance of 70 micrograms could be enough to protect you, he says. The selenium content of foods varies according to the soil in which it was grown. These foods are generally high in selenium — bran, broccoli, cabbage, celery, chicken, cucumbers, eggs, garlic, milk, mushrooms, and wheat germ.

- **Zinc.** Experts have discovered that when prostate tissue becomes cancerous, its zinc levels drop. Coincidence? Probably not. That's why they believe zinc could play a role in keeping your prostate healthy. Though the daily recommended amount of zinc is only 12 to 15 milligrams (mg), experts suggest taking 60 mg for prostate problems. However, taking large doses of zinc can be harmful, so talk with your doctor before taking supplements. A better way might be to eat a handful of pumpkin seeds every day, since they're an outstanding natural source of the mineral.

- **Vitamin D.** Researchers know vitamin D helps prevent prostate cancer. Now, the latest research suggests that vitamin D may even slow the growth of prostate cancer. Since sunlight helps your body produce vitamin D, be sure you spend at least 30 minutes outside every day. To avoid the sun's strongest rays, soak up some sunlight before 10 a.m. and after 4 p.m. Fortified milk is another great way to get vitamin D.

- **Vitamin E.** This powerful antioxidant might also offer some protection against prostate cancer, researchers say. Whole-grain cereals, dark-green vegetables, wheat germ, and nuts are excellent sources.

- **Lycopene.** This seems to be the most promising of the carotenoids, the chemicals that give vegetables their bright orange, yellow, and red colors. Think Italian when you eat — tomatoes and tomato-based products — to add lycopene to your diet.

If you are tempted to take supplements to get some of these nutrients, talk with your doctor before you do, since supplements can have serious side effects.

Spot cancer in your mirror. Men with male pattern baldness (MPB) appear to have a 50-percent higher risk of getting prostate cancer, according to a recent study of almost 4,500 men. MPB could signal cancer decades before more serious symptoms appear. The researchers believe the link might be androgen, a male hormone that could play a role in both conditions. Age and heredity also appear to play a role.

Don't panic if you have less hair on your head than you used to. Just make sure you're up-to-date on your prostate tests.

Get the facts. PSA, or prostate specific antigen, is a protein normally found in your prostate. A PSA screening measures the amount of the compound in your blood in nanograms per milliliter (ng/ml). Having PSA in your blood could signal cancer.

You might not be as current on your prostate screenings as you think. Experts once recommended that most men get their first PSA screening at age 50 and then every year after that. Two new studies suggest otherwise.

All men, according to the new research, should start testing at age 40 and have their second test at age 45. Then, after age 50, your PSA level determines how often you are screened. If you score from zero to 1 ng/ml, then wait three years for your next PSA test. If you score from 1 to 4 ng/ml, then continue testing every year.

As with the old procedure, any score above 4 ng/ml means you are at risk for cancer. The higher the score, the more you're at risk. If this is the case at your next screening, you and your doctor need to discuss further testing and treatment.

Herbal solutions for prostate problems

Herbal remedies might offer as much relief as prescription drugs or surgery for certain prostate conditions. Experts say certain herbs can relieve some of the symptoms of an enlarged prostate. Even more amazing, some herbs are able to treat and prevent cancerous cysts from growing — and a large number of doctors are prescribing them.

Here are some of the more common herbal remedies:

Saw palmetto. By age 60, more than half of all men show signs of benign prostatic hyperplasia (BPH), prostate swelling caused by noncancerous cysts. Simply getting older and being male puts all men at risk. For this natural condition, there's a natural solution. According to several studies, saw palmetto could free you from the symptoms of an enlarged prostate. It appears to help by actually reducing the prostate's size.

Talk with your doctor before taking saw palmetto. If he thinks it's worth a try, visit your local health food store or herb shop. Look for brands that have the ConsumerLabs.com seal of approval on the label.

The recommended dose is 160 milligrams (mg) of extract twice a day or 320 mg once a day. Be patient — it may take several weeks before you notice any improvement.

Pumpkin seeds. In some parts of Europe, men fight BPH every day by munching on a handful of pumpkin seeds. Pumpkin seeds contain cucurbitacins, chemicals that stop testosterone from changing into a stronger form of testosterone, which encourages too many prostate cells to grow. The seeds also contain zinc, a mineral that could reduce the size of your prostate and relieve symptoms of BPH. In one study, a combination of pumpkin seed extract and saw palmetto improved urine flow, relieved painful urination, and significantly reduced the number of times the men needed to urinate during the day and at night.

Talk with your doctor about trying pumpkin seeds. Experts recommend taking two to four teaspoons of ground pumpkin seeds with liquid once in the morning and once at night.

Stinging nettle. In a study including over 140 people, an extract of the stinging nettle plant appeared to stymie the symptoms of BPH without any serious side effects. Stinging nettles grow all across Europe, North America, and maybe even your backyard. But if you want to get some to protect your prostate, visit your local health food store and find the standardized extract of the plant. The recommended daily dose is 150 mg to 300 mg.

African plum tree. As their first defense against prostate problems, Frenchmen take daily doses of the African plum tree, or pygeum. And it seems to work. In one study, two-thirds of the men taking pygeum showed improvements in their symptoms. It might work, according to researchers, because it could reduce prostate inflammation and increase your bladder's output.

PC-SPES. Men suffering from prostate cancer had their prostate specific antigen (PSA) levels decrease by as much as 50 percent or more in two independent studies. For cancer victims, a lower PSA means that their cancer growth could be slowing. The reason for this miracle — a concoction of eight Chinese herbs called PC-SPES. Experts believe PC-SPES acts like the female hormone estrogen, which lowers testosterone levels in men. This weakens cancer's foothold since testosterone seems to encourage tumor growth.

However promising it might sound, this herbal potion won't prevent prostate cancer. Instead, PC-SPES seems to be best for cancer victims who have tried all other medications and have nothing to lose. It seems especially beneficial for men with androgen-independent cancer, since that type of prostate cancer is resistant to most other medications. Experts also warn against everyday PC-SPES use because it could cause serious side effects, like blood clots and impotency.

PSORIASIS

Psoriasis self-help made easy

If you want something done right, do it yourself. That seems to be the philosophy of many people with psoriasis. According to the National Psoriasis Foundation (NPF), self-treatment is becoming more popular for people with this skin condition.

You can choose from a variety of alternative remedies ranging from acupuncture to magnets. However, there's little scientific evidence that any of these therapies work. To help make your choice of treatments easier, here are some of the more effective and proven psoriasis self-help strategies.

Hit the beach. This sounds too fun to be therapy, but it's true. Spending some time in the sun and water — a strategy called "climatotherapy" — offers relief to many people with psoriasis. In fact, according to the NPF, 80 percent of those who get regular exposure to the sun show improvement. It's the sun's ultraviolet light that helps clear up your skin.

> ### What is it?
>
> With this chronic condition, your skin cells multiply much faster than normal and build up into scaly, red, and irritated patches called plaques. They can appear on your scalp, elbows, palms, soles, and knees, as well as in the folds of your skin.
>
> Symptoms:
> - Red, thick patches or sores
> - Silvery scales
> - Itchiness
> - Dryness
> - Inflamed, painful skin
> - Arthritis

If you're nowhere near a beach, that's OK. Dr. Steven R. Feldman, a professor of dermatology and pathology at Wake Forest University School of Medicine, recommends an easy solution.

"Of the alternative treatments, the most effective is tanning beds... since we know how good ultraviolet light is for psoriasis," Feldman says. "Sunny beach vacations are also outstanding."

Not to mention more fun. The most popular location for psoriasis treatment is the Dead Sea, which offers plenty of sunlight and special water. But traveling halfway around the world might not be the most practical approach.

Don't worry — you can get the benefit of "climatotherapy" at the Jersey shore or any beach near you. Just make sure you sunbathe safely, because too much exposure to the sun can cause skin cancer. Ask your dermatologist about any precautions you should take — such as using sunscreen and avoiding the sun at its peak hours of 10 a.m. to 2 p.m. And enjoy your day in the sun.

Chill out. Stress doesn't only aggravate you — it also aggravates your psoriasis. One good way to keep your psoriasis in check is to keep your stress levels under control.

Studies have shown that hypnosis and relaxation tapes help conventional treatments work even better. But anything that helps the mind relax comes in handy. Try stress management techniques such as yoga, tai chi, or meditation. Exercise often cuts down on stress, too. However you do it, relax. It will only make things better.

Go fish. Many supplements claim to fight psoriasis. One that actually works is fish oil. In several clinical trials, fish oil supplements improved the symptoms of psoriasis, including scales, redness, and itching. As a bonus, fish oil also helps boost your mood, improve your memory, and defend against heart attacks and strokes. Another supplement possibly worth trying is evening primrose oil, which helped relieve other skin disorders in a number of studies.

The fatty acids in these supplements protect your skin and fight inflammation, which might have something to do with psoriasis. Just talk to your doctor before taking any supplements.

Rub it in. To treat psoriasis, you need to moisturize your skin. A wide range of topical products — those you apply to your skin — might do the trick. Aloe vera helped treat psoriasis in one study, and other natural over-the-counter moisturizing products could be effective. Bath products that contain oats soothe the skin, while products containing capsaicin helped clear up scaly skin, redness, and itching in some studies. One of the oldest remedies for psoriasis is coal tar, which you can get with or without a prescription. You should probably use it under a doctor's supervision, though.

Feldman says a combination of a strong cortisone-type medication and an ointment called Dovonex, a substance similar to vitamin D, is the best way to clear psoriasis for those with only a few spots. Ask your doctor about these prescription medications.

"In most cases, it's probably a good idea to see a dermatologist to confirm the diagnosis and to establish a treatment plan," Feldman says. He also believes it's important to quit smoking, stop excessive drinking, eat a healthy diet, and exercise regularly.

"Even if these don't help the psoriasis, they are still a good idea," he notes. "Especially the alcohol part, because alcohol can damage the liver, and some of the best medicines for psoriasis can't be used in people with damaged livers."

Don't let psoriasis get under your skin

When you have psoriasis, you're dealing with more than meets the eye. Along with the physical symptoms comes a complex mix of emotions. Sheri Decker should know — she's had psoriasis for 31 years.

"The feelings you have because of psoriasis can run the gamut from anger, frustration, sadness, despair, guilt, shame, bewilderment, exasperation, and even acceptance," says Decker, director of communications for the National Psoriasis Foundation.

Meet the challenge of severe psoriasis

One severe but little-known form of psoriasis is psoriatic arthritis. This painful condition, whose cause remains unknown, develops in 10 to 30 percent of people with psoriasis.

Psoriatic arthritis can occur at any age but usually strikes between the ages of 30 and 50. Along with the scaly spots that normally come with psoriasis, symptoms include joint pain, swelling, and stiffness; fingernail and toenail lesions; trouble moving; sausage-like look to fingers and toes; and eye redness and pain.

Besides the usual remedies for psoriasis, you can use these treatments for psoriatic arthritis:

- ↪ **Exercise.** Keep up your strength and mobility. Stretching is especially important.
- ↪ **Rest.** Take a break to ease the pain.
- ↪ **Heat and cold.** Use these treatments to relieve pain and reduce swelling.
- ↪ **Splints.** Support an aching joint so you can move — and feel — better.
- ↪ **Medications.** Aspirin and other nonsteroidal anti-inflammatory drugs (NSAIDs) soothe inflammation and joint pain. Disease-modifying anti-rheumatic drugs (DMARDs) tackle more severe symptoms and stop your condition from getting worse.
- ↪ **Surgery.** This might be necessary in extreme cases.

"You may experience any of these emotions at different times. For example, you can go from feeling despair to acceptance and then to anger. The feelings seem to wax and wane over time, just as the physical symptoms of the disease often do."

Just as important as it is to take care of your skin, it's equally important to deal with your negative emotions. Don't despair. You can overcome the bad feelings by taking the following steps.

Talk openly about your condition. Don't be ashamed of it. It's not your fault. You don't need to come up with elaborate lies about being burned or injured. Explain psoriasis — and stress that it's not contagious — to people who may not know anything about it. Chances are they'll be interested. You'll help educate people and possibly make new friends.

You might not feel comfortable talking about psoriasis right away, but practice makes perfect. Anticipate questions people might ask (or want to ask) and prepare responses. Do this until you no longer feel awkward talking about it.

Join forces with others. Support groups where you share feelings and experiences can help tremendously. If nothing else, you'll realize you're not alone. Other people with psoriasis are going through the same emotions you are, and that knowledge may help you banish those negative feelings.

The National Psoriasis Foundation sponsors a Pen Pal Club to put people with psoriasis in touch with each other. But you don't have to limit your activities to groups of people with psoriasis. Just being involved with other people can make a difference.

"It is OK to feel sad, angry, or depressed, but you need to work through those emotions," Decker says. "You will need the support of other people. Don't go it alone."

Focus on your own feelings. In other words, worry only about how you feel, not what strangers think of you. It's difficult because, whether we admit it or not, other people's opinions make a difference. So it hurts when they move away from you at restaurants and beaches or ask you to leave a public swimming pool. But if you're comfortable with yourself, you'll be better equipped to shrug off ignorant comments or dirty looks.

"Once someone gets psoriasis, they have to relearn to live in society marked as different, and this is a difficult task," Decker says. "It is important that you realize you will have emotional responses because of psoriasis, because once you do, then you can deal with them."

If your feelings become overwhelming, don't hesitate to seek professional help.

Learn the facts. Arm yourself with information about psoriasis. You can find plenty of valuable materials from the National Psoriasis Foundation. Besides keeping you informed, they will help remind you that you have a medical problem, not some bizarre curse.

"I think knowledge is the most important tool in overcoming negative emotions," Decker says. "Learn as much as you can about psoriasis. Learn the facts and what is scientifically known about psoriasis. Avoid the myths and speculation about what might have caused it and what might cure it."

Put it in perspective. Of course, you're not going to be happy all the time. But try to keep focused on positive things — your family, friends, job, hobbies, whatever you find important.

Don't let psoriasis dominate your life. It will always be a part of your life, for sure — but remember it's not the only part.

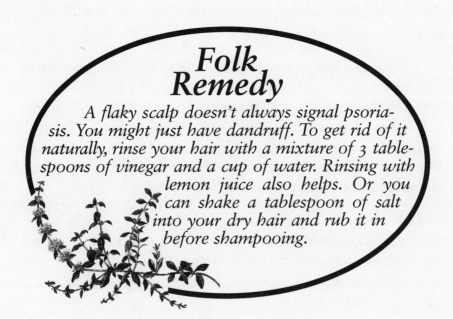

Folk
Remedy

A flaky scalp doesn't always signal psoriasis. You might just have dandruff. To get rid of it naturally, rinse your hair with a mixture of 3 tablespoons of vinegar and a cup of water. Rinsing with lemon juice also helps. Or you can shake a tablespoon of salt into your dry hair and rub it in before shampooing.

RHEUMATOID ARTHRITIS

Lowering your risk

Why does one sister in a family fall prey to crippling rheumatoid arthritis (RA) while her siblings remain healthy? No one can say for sure just yet, but researchers are discovering that certain risk factors can make you more vulnerable to this autoimmune disease. Some of those risks lie out of your control, but you can avoid others with lifestyle changes.

Female. Experts think female hormones have something to do with the development of RA. That's because several autoimmune diseases — including RA — show up more often in women than men. But after menopause, when hormone levels decrease, the difference is not as great.

Smoking. Scientists recently found a connection between RA and women who smoke. According to their study,

What is it?

This common type of arthritis affects your entire body. For some unknown reason, your immune system attacks healthy joints, causing the lining to swell. If left untreated, rheumatoid arthritis can permanently damage bone and cartilage and can even spread to some of your internal organs.

Symptoms:
- Swollen, stiff, warm, painful joints
- Loss of appetite and energy
- Fever
- Anemia
- Knobby, disfigured joints

289

the risk was highest for women who smoked the most cigarettes for the greatest number of years. On average, current female smokers had nearly twice the risk of having RA as women who never smoked. The risk of former smokers was higher than in women who never smoked, but not nearly as high as current smokers. If you want to reduce your chances of getting this devastating disease, throw out your cigarettes today. You could be saving yourself from a lifetime of disability.

Coffee. Could that pot of coffee you brew and drink each day be putting you at risk for RA? Researchers in Finland think it might be. Their study suggested that people who drink four or more cups of coffee a day more than doubled their risk of getting a type of RA in which rheumatoid factor is present in the blood. Positive rheumatoid factor often signals a worse course for those with the disease. More research is necessary, however, because most of the people studied in Finland drank boiled coffee — a method of preparation you probably don't use. Future studies will consider other ways coffee is prepared, since today most people use automatic coffee makers. Meanwhile, it makes sense to limit your coffee drinking to a few cups a day.

Bacteria. In the early part of the 20th century, there was talk of infections causing rheumatoid arthritis. Over the years, a few doctors tried treating patients with antibiotics — with some good results. But most doctors didn't buy the theory that RA could be reversed with antibiotics, and they continued to search for new drugs to make their patients more comfortable. A new study could change all that. Researchers in Israel recently found evidence of a bacterium called *mycoplasma fermentans* in the fluid surrounding the joints of RA sufferers. The finding caught the medical world's attention because scientists know mycoplasmas can cause arthritis in animals. The researchers think mycoplasmas in your joints start a chain reaction of inflammation and tissue damage.

With the renewed focus on infection, antibiotics might soon be a common treatment for RA.

Creative ways to cope with RA

Coping with the pain and exhaustion of rheumatoid arthritis (RA) can be overwhelming — even with prescription medicine. Fortunately, strong medicine isn't your only resource. Many people find relief with alternative remedies. Try these drug-free ways of dealing with RA.

Use that old-time religion. When 35 people with RA kept diaries for a study, researchers learned spirituality can be a key to coping with pain. The people who had daily spiritual experiences — such as being moved by the beauty of creation — were in better moods and had much less joint pain. These people were also more likely to have a support group to help them when things got rough. Don't let the stress of RA keep you from tuning in to your spiritual side. Stay involved with a group of like-minded people, and your body could profit along with your spirit.

Intensify exercise. You're probably tempted to baby your joints after an RA flare, but experts say you should do just the opposite. In a recent study, people hospitalized for RA were put on a program of muscle strengthening exercises five times a week and bicycle conditioning three times a week in addition to their usual range-of-motion exercises. Another group simply did the range-of-motion exercises. After 24 weeks, the super exercisers had much better muscle strength and were functioning better physically. Ask your doctor about cranking up your exercise program. You might be capable of more than you think.

Keep moving. Have you been skipping your workouts because you'll just have to quit when your RA flares? Keep up the workouts in between, experts say, and you'll do better in the long run. Researchers found that people who backed off on exercise after they had a flare-up felt more upset about their disease and more limited by it as time went on. Stay tough mentally, and don't let RA rob you of any activities without a fight. Even though you have to rest your joints during a flare, get back into action as soon as you are able.

If you need direction and motivation, ask your doctor about physical therapy. In a recent study, people with moderate to severe RA had physical therapists come to their homes for six weeks to teach them about exercise. Another group with similar symptoms did nothing different. After 12 weeks, the group that received physical therapy had fewer tender joints, less morning stiffness, and better grip strength. And a follow-up study done a year later revealed that the results were long lasting.

Indulge in a massage. Who wouldn't enjoy a soothing rub-down? It can loosen tight muscles and help you relax — two things you need when you have RA. If you don't have someone at home who can give you a massage, ask your doctor to recommend a professional. For a real treat, visit a day spa that offers massage. You'll feel pampered and renewed by the time you leave. Just be careful of joints that are painful or inflamed since massage can make them worse.

Get needled. Acupuncture, which has been around for thousands of years, requires a trained professional to place sterile needles in various parts of your body. Usually the acupuncturist leaves them in for about 20 minutes. Acupressure is similar, but it's done with pressure, not needles. Although the jury is still out on whether or not these practices work, many people claim they've gotten long-lasting relief. If you'd like to try something different, check with your doctor first, then find a licensed acupuncturist or acupressurist. With a little luck, you might even be able to find a medical doctor who performs this service.

Help yourself with herbs. Although using herbal supplements for RA is still controversial, some have been used for centuries with good results.

- **Bromelain and boswellia.** Scott Zashin, one of the best medical doctors in the country, according to the authors of *Best Doctors in America*, uses conventional and alternative therapies in his practice in Texas. For his RA patients, he sometimes recommends bromelain and boswellia. He says they may reduce inflammation. Bromelain is an enzyme that occurs naturally in pineapple. You can buy bromelain extract in capsules at health food stores and herb shops. The usual dosage is 400 to 600 mg three times a day. Boswellia, also known as frankincense, is used in India as a traditional remedy for rheumatic inflammation. It can slow down inflammation and increase blood supply to your joints. The usual dosage is 150 mg of the extract three times a day.

- **Tripterygium.** This plant, used in China to treat autoimmune diseases, is also known as "thunder god vine." Studies show it works by partially blocking inflammation. In a 12-week study, people with RA and their doctors said they saw a significant improvement in the participants taking tripterygium compared with a sugar pill.

Soothing relief from oil

If your arthritic joints feel like rusty hinges, maybe it's time to oil them — from the inside. Studies show that certain oils from fish and plants can improve rheumatoid arthritis (RA) symptoms

Has researcher found cure for RA?

Until recently, the only hope for rheumatoid arthritis sufferers was stronger drugs to help with discomfort and inflammation. But now a professor in London thinks he may have found the key to curing RA.

Dr. Jonathan Edwards of University College tried removing faulty B lymphocytes — a type of white blood cell — from people with RA. He guessed that would allow normal lymphocytes to grow in their place. So far, it looks like he was right.

Instead of doing their job of keeping disease away, RA sufferers' B lymphocytes attack joints as though they were the enemy.

Edwards gave drugs specially designed to kill off the trouble-making cells to five women with RA. Two women needed treatment more than once, but all five showed dramatic improvement. After a year and a half, three of the women had no tender joints, and the other two women had only one or two.

Researchers are now working on a larger trial of the therapy, which involves a short stay in the hospital. If all goes well, this exciting new treatment could be available to the public in a few years.

by reducing inflammation, the cause of much RA pain. Although research is still ongoing, it looks like dietary oils could be an important part of preventing and fighting this painful disease. Here's where you can find these valuable oils.

Fish. Eskimos rarely get arthritis. Experts say it's because they eat lots of cold-water fish loaded with omega-3 oils, which help fight inflammation. In fact, a recent study found that women who ate one or two servings of broiled or baked fish a week were less likely to get RA than women who didn't eat fish.

While studying arthritis in rats, Jaya Venkatraman, Ph.D., a professor at the State University of New York at Buffalo, discovered that fish oils combined with vitamin E could reduce pain and swelling. She knew that molecules called cytokines played a role in inflammation, although not all cytokines cause trouble. But in rheumatoid arthritis, certain cytokines multiply out of control, making your joints swell and hurt.

Somehow, fish oil sends helpful cytokines to the rescue. "... The combination of fish oil, with its omega-3 fatty acids, and vitamin E," Venkatraman says, "appears to help restore the balance between pro- and anti-inflammatory cytokines. It probably can't prevent development of rheumatoid arthritis, but it may delay symptoms and allow a reduction in other medication. People who normally had to take 10 aspirins a day, for example, may be able to take five. This therapy also seems to improve function."

Two or three times each week eat fatty fish, such as salmon, mackerel, albacore tuna, bluefish, anchovies, or herring. Be sure to buy fish caught in the ocean, not from fish farms, which produce fish lower in omega-3. You might not notice results for several months, so hang in there.

If eating that much fish makes you queasy, you can buy fish oil in capsules, but check with your doctor first. The oil can affect how your blood clots, and it can interfere with certain medications. Once you get the go-ahead, be sure to buy a reputable brand. Researchers recommend taking 3 to 5 grams of oil a day for best results. Some people find fish oil so helpful they are able to cut back on nonsteroidal anti-inflammatory drugs (NSAIDs).

Vitamin E. This vitamin is a powerful antioxidant, capable of defending your body against destructive free radicals that can weaken your immune system. Because RA is considered an autoimmune disease, scientists are starting to look at how antioxidants might help boost your immune system. One study found that people with RA had evidence of increased free radicals at work but, at the same time, lower levels of vitamin E than other people. If you increase your vitamin E intake, you might prevent some of the tissue damage caused by RA. You can find this antioxidant in wheat germ oil, sunflower seeds, almonds, avocados, brown rice, safflower oil, and dry roasted peanuts.

Pumpkin seed oil. This nut-flavored oil, extracted from pumpkin seeds, is a folk remedy for many ailments. It fights inflammation thanks to its combination of omega-3 fatty acids, vitamin E, and other antioxidants. When animals with arthritis were given pumpkin seed oil, swelling decreased by 44 percent — an amount researchers called remarkable. You can use it for cooking and in salad dressings. Also known as "green gold" because of its color, the oil comes from Austria. If you can't find it at your grocery or health food store, you can order it online from an Austrian company called Green Gold. According to their Web site, you can use the oil for up to one year. For more information, go to <www.greengold.net>.

Olive oil. What could be more delicious than freshly cooked vegetables topped with zesty olive oil and a dash of salt? How about knowing that you're eating away at your pain, too? A recent study in Greece found that the more fresh vegetables and olive oil people ate, the less likely they were to get RA. Of course, it's possible that fish eaten in a typical Greek diet affected the results. So keep eating fish and start pouring olive oil on your salads and cooked vegetables, and you'll cover all your bases.

Evening primrose oil. Researchers aren't sure why this oil helps relieve painful RA since it's made primarily of omega-6 oils instead of omega-3. They think it might be competing with molecules that cause inflammation. What they do know is that evening primrose oil works for many RA sufferers.

Flaxseed oil. The flax plant was used for thousands of years, both for food and for making linen. It has been replaced in modern times by oils that stay fresh longer. After fish, flaxseed oil is the next best source of omega-3 fatty acids. Researchers found that a diet high in flaxseed oil reduces the out-of-control cytokines that cause inflammation — just like fish. For every 100 pounds of your body weight, experts recommend taking one tablespoon of flaxseed oil daily. It has an earthy, almost fishy taste. If you can't take it straight, try disguising it on salads and vegetables. To keep flaxseed oil fresh, store it in your refrigerator or freezer. It's definitely worth the trouble.

Thwart related diseases with early detection

The damaging effects of arthritis could harm more than your joints. You're also at increased risk for other diseases, such as heart disease and osteoporosis. Fortunately, if you know what you're dealing with, you'll have a better chance of fending them off and staying healthy.

Heart disease. Scientists are still debating why having RA puts you at greater risk for heart disease, but in the meantime, they've made a few educated guesses. Some think it's because people with limited movement tend to gain weight and avoid exercise — two known risk factors for heart disease. So it makes sense to keep your weight down and stay as active as possible.

Unfortunately, it's not that simple. Studies show that people with RA often have high cholesterol and high triglyceride levels that have nothing to do with their weight. And high cholesterol and triglycerides also increase heart disease risk. Another study points to the inflammation that goes hand in hand with autoimmune diseases, like RA. Inflammation can damage your heart, another reason why people with RA are more likely to have heart problems.

If you have RA, experts recommend eating a low-fat diet and exercising several times a week. Your doctor should check your cholesterol and triglyceride levels regularly, and if they're high, you might need to take medicine to help bring them down.

Taking steroids long-term for your RA can cause high blood pressure and raise your "bad" cholesterol. Talk with your doctor about new prescription drugs that can reduce inflammation and protect your heart as well.

Osteoporosis. Women with RA are twice as likely as other women to develop this bone-thinning disease. Researchers say taking corticosteroids, being thin, and avoiding physical activity can all contribute to bone thinning. In addition, having positive rheumatoid factor in your blood — something many people with RA have — increases your risk. In spite of this, you don't have to resign yourself to weak bones.

The American College of Rheumatology recommends steroid users take the following measures to avoid osteoporosis.

 ⊸ Take the lowest effective dose of steroid you can.

 ⊸ Don't smoke.

 ⊸ Strive for a healthy weight for your frame.

 ⊸ Keep alcohol to a minimum.

 ⊸ Do weight-bearing exercises 30 to 60 minutes a day and any exercises recommended by your doctor or physical therapist.

 ⊸ Have a bone density scan when you begin steroid therapy and then every six months to one year to compare results.

 ⊸ Consider hormone replacement therapy or other medications that help prevent osteoporosis if you're post-menopausal.

↪ Get 1,500 mg of calcium and 800 IU of vitamin D each day.

Sjögren's. This drying syndrome typically affects the eyes and mouth, but it can also affect other parts of your body that have moisture-producing glands, such as your nose and throat. If you have Sjögren's, you might experience a burning sensation in your tongue or throat; lung or kidney problems; gritty eyes; tooth decay; or dry skin. At this time, there is no known cure for

---

Avoid these dangerous combinations

If you want to take supplements for your arthritis or another condition, always check with your doctor first. Certain supplements can interact with your medication, and you could find yourself with new health problems. Here are some examples.

↪ **Ginger.** Herbal experts recommend ginger for arthritis, but watch out if you're taking medicine, too. Ginger can strengthen the effects of anticoagulants such as heparin, warfarin, and ticlopidine. By keeping your blood less sticky, ginger raises the odds of bleeding.

↪ **Garlic.** Like ginger, garlic keeps your blood from clumping or clotting. It can lead to bleeding when taken along with blood-thinning medications like warfarin or ticlopidine.

↪ **Ginkgo.** People take ginkgo for circulation problems and to sharpen thinking. But your blood pressure could shoot up if you're also taking thiazide diuretics. You might also have bleeding problems if you're taking heparin or warfarin.

↪ **Oil supplements.** Arthritis sufferers often take fish oil or other oil supplements to reduce inflammation. In rare cases, oils react to medicine. Fish oil, borage oil, and evening primrose oil could trigger bruising and nosebleeds if taken with aspirin or other nonsteroidal anti-inflammatory drugs (NSAIDs), such as ibuprofen or naproxen.

Sjögren's syndrome, but you can make yourself more comfortable with the following tips:

- ✦ Try a saliva substitute. Look for one approved by the American Dental Association. You can also buy over-the-counter tablets that help stimulate saliva.

- ✦ Chew gum containing the sugar substitute Xylitol, which naturally stimulates saliva.

- ✦ Sip milk. It can help keep your mouth moistened and prevent tooth decay.

- ✦ Have your eyes examined often and buy artificial teardrops to keep your eyes moist. Eyes that are constantly dry and gritty can become infected easily.

- ✦ Wear sunglasses outdoors and don't use contact lenses.

- ✦ Try a humidifier in your home to keep your eyes, mouth, and nose from feeling dry.

Scleritis. This ongoing inflammation of the blood vessels of the whites of your eyes causes pain and redness. It's serious because it can cause permanent damage if not treated early. If the whites of your eyes are red and painful, see an ophthalmologist immediately. Prompt treatment with special eye drops or anti-inflammatory drugs could save your sight.

Outsmart ticks to prevent achy joints

Your joints have been aching so badly lately you can't even muster the strength to play golf — your favorite outdoor activity. If you think getting older is causing your joints to ache, think again. Your age might not be the problem. Something may be lurking on the golf course that's causing your aches and pains.

Elyes Zhioua, a researcher from the University of Rhode Island, found the edges of golf courses in Rhode Island teeming with ticks infected with the bacteria that cause Lyme disease. In fact, on some golf courses, up to 75 percent of ticks he tested carried the bacteria.

Lyme disease can develop after an infected tick bite. If left untreated, it can cause severe headaches, heart problems, and arthritis. Although you are most likely to encounter infected ticks in the Northeast or Mid-Atlantic region, Lyme disease has surfaced in 47 states so far.

You don't have to stay inside to protect yourself — just remember to take a few precautions before you venture out.

- **Seal yourself off.** Experts recommend you wear pants and long sleeves when walking in tall grass or the woods. Tuck your shirt into your pants and pull your socks over your pants to seal off as much of your skin as possible. Use insect repellent that claims it will keep ticks away. Pull your hair back if it's long and wear a hat.

- **Check regularly.** Get in the habit of checking yourself and others in your family for ticks. Look carefully in favorite tick hiding places — folds of skin and hair. If you do find a tick, don't panic or pull it off with your fingers. If it's not attached, go outdoors and brush it off with a stiff piece of paper. Lyme disease doesn't usually develop unless an infected tick has been attached to you for at least 36 hours. If you do find one attached, gently pull it out with tweezers, grasping it from its head area. Don't pull at the middle of the tick. That could make it burst and spread bacteria. After removing a tick, swab the area with an antiseptic.

- **Know the signs.** Not every tick carries the bacteria for Lyme disease. But watch for a spreading rash shaped like a bull's-eye after a tick bite, a symptom in 80 percent of people who test positive for the disease. You might also experience fever, headache, a stiff neck, and joint pain but not everybody has all of these symptoms before getting the disease. If you suspect you may have been infected, see your doctor. He can do a blood test to decide if you need antibiotics. Research shows that people who get antibiotics soon after infection are less likely to develop arthritis symptoms.

↦ **Consider getting the vaccine.** The FDA recently approved a vaccine that can reduce your chances of getting Lyme disease by about 80 percent. If you're between the ages of 15 and 70, live in the Northeast or Mid-Atlantic area, and spend a good deal of time outdoors, this might be a good option.

Folk Remedy

Ancient Egyptians had a stylish cure for arthritis — copper jewelry. Even today, some people claim that wearing a piece of copper against your skin allows your body to absorb this essential mineral and fight arthritis.

While experts say it's possible that a copper deficiency contributes to rheumatoid arthritis, there's no proof that copper jewelry helps. But it doesn't seem to hurt, either. Besides, you might enjoy looking like Cleopatra.

ROSACEA

Proven ways to relieve rosacea

Legendary comedian W.C. Fields had rosacea, but this condition is no laughing matter.

Rosacea often strikes in your 30s and 40s, but it may be just as common — and more severe — after age 50. Women and people with fair complexions get rosacea more often, but it can affect anyone. It also attacks men and women differently. Signs of rosacea normally show up on women's cheeks and chins, while the nose — like that of Fields — becomes the target area for men.

Although rosacea has no cure, you can take steps to manage this chronic disease. Make a plan for living with rosacea.

Find your triggers. First, you have to discover what sparks your rosacea flare-ups. Triggers can vary from cold or hot weather to spicy foods, alcohol, or hot baths. In short, anything that makes your face flush is a potential trigger. One person with rosacea might get flare-ups from salsa, while another can eat salsa but flushes from

---

What is it?

Rosacea is a chronic disease that affects the skin of your face. It begins with a frequent flushing of your cheeks, similar to a blush or sunburn. Eventually, areas of your face become permanently red. You may develop an acne-like rash, as well.

It's not clear what causes rosacea. Triggers include hot or spicy foods, alcohol, stress, extreme temperatures, menopause, and certain medicines. Rosacea cannot be cured, but it can be treated.

Symptoms:
- Redness
- Pimples
- Enlarged facial blood vessels
- Red, bumpy nose
- Swelling of the nose

---

drinking wine. Therefore, you don't have to give up everything — just the things that aggravate your rosacea. Keeping a diary to track your flare-ups might help.

Then, once you've determined your personal triggers, make some lifestyle changes to cope with rosacea.

Modify your diet. What you eat and drink has a big impact on your rosacea. Besides spicy foods and alcohol, other common culprits include liver, yogurt, cheese, soy sauce, vinegar, sour cream, citrus fruits, chocolate, vanilla, eggplant, spinach, avocados, hot chocolate, coffee, and tea.

"Diet seems very important," says Dr. Joel Bamford, a dermatologist at St. Mary's-Duluth Health System in Minnesota. "A lot of our patients who had rosacea associated theirs with dairy products. You probably don't want to eat a lot of hot liquids or foods. The temperature of food makes them flush. It's a normal thing; it's just more obvious for people with rosacea."

Partly because of Fields' trademark bulbous nose and constant references to drinking, rosacea is often incorrectly linked to alcoholism. In reality, teetotalers can suffer from it just as much. But alcohol does aggravate the condition for many people.

If you do have one too many drinks — or too much chocolate or whatever else triggers your rosacea — and have a flushing episode, Bamford suggests chewing on ice chips for relief.

Protect your skin. It's important to take care of your face. When washing your face, stay away from harsh, grainy soaps and rough washcloths. Use a gentle, fragrance-free cleanser instead. Rinse with lukewarm water and gently blot your face dry with a soft towel. Once your face is dry, apply your medication. Then you can put on some moisturizer or camouflaging make-up. Green-tinted foundation helps some people offset the red.

Make sure to use sunscreen, even on overcast days. If it irritates your face, try a brand made for children. These are usually gentler. Don't go outside in the heat between 10 a.m. and 2 p.m., when the sun is at its strongest. Wear a scarf or ski mask in the winter to protect your face from the cold and wind.

Handle your emotions. A recent survey of 700 people with rosacea by the National Rosacea Society found that for 91 percent of them, emotional stress led to flare-ups. Most common kinds of stress included anxiety, anger, frustration, worry, and embarrassment.

"People call attention to your appearance, so that's embarrassing, and a reason for being more flushed," Bamford says. "And stress can make one flush and contribute to the appearance of rosacea."

Family, jobs, finances, health, relationships, and social pressure caused the most stress. The good news is 83 percent of those surveyed who tried stress management said it helped keep rosacea flare-ups in check.

Bamford suggests deciding if the problem is stress-related first, then coming up with a strategy to deal with the situation. One option, of course, is to avoid what's causing the stress. Another is to talk to a friend, minister, or even a psychologist.

"There's also biofeedback, meditation, tai chi," Bamford adds, noting that each person must figure out what works best for them. "It's such a personal thing, what you do about stress."

Exercise is a great way to work out stress, but don't overdo it. Sometimes during heavy exercise, you become too flushed and bring on a flare-up. Explore different relaxation techniques to see what works for you. You'll stop seeing red — literally.

Ulcer cure may save your skin

Want to understand rosacea better? Maybe you should take a look at your stomach.

Although rosacea has no known cause, a link has been suggested between the skin condition and *Helicobacter pylori*. This type of bacterium, more commonly called *H. pylori*, has already been linked to stomach problems such as gastritis and ulcers.

Some researchers have found that *H. pylori* appears in people with rosacea and that treating *H. pylori* helps clear up the rosacea. They conclude the stomach bug has something to do with the skin disorder. But, as you'll see, that theory has quite a few bugs of its own.

Examine the research. Dr. Alfredo Rebora, an Italian dermatologist, originally proposed the link between *H. pylori* and rosacea.

"Dr. Rebora in Italy noticed a lot of his patients had *helicobacter* and also had rosacea," says Dr. Joel Bamford, a dermatologist at St. Mary's-Duluth Health System in Minnesota. But, adds Bamford, he didn't take into account that many people in Italy (not just those with rosacea) had *H. pylori*.

In several parts of the world — for example, Paraguay and certain areas of Russia — an astounding 95 percent of the people have the bacteria in their systems, according to Bamford. That compares to a rate of about 15 percent in the United States, he says.

Studies in Turkey and Poland found *H. pylori* is present in some people with rosacea and that treating the *H. pylori* also cleared their skin. But rather than prove a definite link, these studies just add to the speculation. The Turkish study, in particular, has drawn criticism from other researchers because of its poor methods and design.

Look at the evidence. Less questionable studies have disputed the relationship between *H. pylori* and rosacea.

Bamford and others from the St. Mary's-Duluth Health System found no link between the bacteria and the skin condition. In that study, half of the 44 subjects were treated for *H. pylori* and the other half were given a placebo, or dummy, treatment. Both groups showed the same improvement in rosacea symptoms. In other words, treating *H. pylori* was no more effective in relieving rosacea symptoms than doing virtually nothing. A more recent Korean study reached the same conclusion.

Another study at the University of South Carolina determined that *H. pylori* is no more common in people with rosacea than in those without the condition. However, more people with rosacea did complain of indigestion (which had nothing to do with *H. pylori*) and take antacids.

Consider the cure. One explanation for the pro-link results in some studies lies in the antibiotics used to knock out *H. pylori*.

"The same antibiotics used to treat *helicobacter* are used to suppress rosacea," Bamford explains. "It makes sense if you treat someone for *helicobacter*, they get temporary improvement in rosacea."

So, while there's no solid reason to suspect a link between *H. pylori* and rosacea, there may still be a good reason to go after rosacea with antibiotics. Ask your doctor about using an oral or topical antibiotic to treat your skin condition.

Lose the heat but not the flavor

You might have to give up spicy seasonings like pepper, paprika, and cayenne because of your rosacea, but that doesn't mean you have to hand over your taste buds. Instead, swap these zesty recipes from the National Rosacea Society for typical spicy condiments.

Instead of	Try
Chili powder	2 tsp cumin and 1 tsp oregano
Poultry seasoning	1/2 tsp sage, 1/2 tsp coriander, 1/4 tsp thyme, 1/8 tsp allspice, and 1/8 tsp marjoram
Curry powder	4 tsp coriander, 2 tsp turmeric, 1 tsp cinnamon, 1 tsp cumin, 1/2 tsp basil or oregano, and 1/2 tsp cardamom

SKIN CANCER

Get the 'skin'ny on sunscreen

Wearing sunscreen — incorrectly — could put you at risk for melanoma, the deadliest type of skin cancer. If you don't choose the right sunscreen or apply it properly, your skin is in as much danger as if you weren't wearing sunscreen at all.

The whole reason for sunscreen is to protect you from the sun's two types of scorching rays — ultraviolet A (UVA) and ultraviolet B (UVB). Both suppress your immune system and can cause skin cancer. Most sunscreens only block UVB rays, so, for protection from UVA rays, buy products labeled as "broad spectrum" sunscreens.

Make sunscreen a part of your daily routine, like brushing your teeth or combing your hair. And learn the where, when, and how of good sun sense.

Know your SPF. According to the American Academy of Dermatology (AAD), the Sun Protection Factor, or SPF, is a number that refers to the product's ability to block out

---

What is it?

Cancerous cells in the outer layers of your skin affect over a million people every year. There are three types — basal cell carcinoma, squamous cell carcinoma, and malignant melanoma. Melanoma is the most deadly, but it is also the least common.

Symptoms:
- Irregularly-shaped moles
- A red, scaly patch of skin
- Moles larger than a pencil eraser
- Multi-colored moles
- Any change in a mole's appearance
- Sores that don't heal

the sun's burning rays. It is figured by comparing the amount of time it takes to burn protected skin, to the amount of time it takes to burn unprotected skin. For instance, if you sunburn without sunscreen in 10 minutes, it would take 150 minutes to burn if you were wearing a sunscreen with SPF 15.

Sunscreen products range from SPF 2 to SPF 60, however, most dermatologists believe an SPF of less than 4 is not really even a sunscreen and anything over 30 offers little added benefit. The AAD recommends an SPF of at least 15 for everyone, but go for higher protection if you:

- have a light complexion.

- have ever had skin cancer in the past.

- have a family member who had skin cancer.

If you have a serious illness or are on medication, talk with your doctor before spending any length of time in the sun.

Don't skimp. One of the biggest mistakes you can make, experts say, is not putting enough sunscreen on. To get the coverage you need, the average adult should use about one ounce of sunscreen — that's the amount it takes to fill a shot glass.

Plan ahead. It takes 20 to 30 minutes for sunscreen to soak into your skin. So, slather on the lotion well before going outside. This will also give it time to dry so it won't rub off on your clothes or your car seat.

Watch the clock. While a good sunscreen is critical for skin protection, many people believe a high SPF sunscreen means it's safe to stay in the sun longer. This probably explains why people who use a high factor sunscreen still get sunburned.

Whatever your SPF choice, experts suggest you keep sun exposure to small doses and reapply sunscreen every two hours.

Rinse and repeat. Going to the beach or pool means extra sunburn risk. Most swimmers will get burned despite the fact they use sunscreen. Even waterproof sunscreens come off after swimming and toweling dry. Play it safe and apply more when you come out of the water.

Don't bug out. Let's say you're bothered by bugs AND the sun. An insect repellent containing DEET will fend off the creepy-crawlies, but will make your sunscreen a third less effective. On the other hand, a product containing both sunscreen and insect repellent seems to hold off the sun, but not the bugs. You choose which is more important for your outing and take extra precautions, if necessary.

Keep an eye on the index. The National Weather Service and the Environmental Protection Agency (EPA) together developed a scale — from 0 to 10 — to let people know how much UV radiation reaches the Earth at any given time. It's called a UV Index. Use it to decide how much sun protection you'll need for the day.

UV Index Number	UV Radiation Exposure
0-2	minimal
3-4	low
5-6	moderate
7-9	high
10+	very high

You can find the UV Index with your newspaper's weather map, or on the local television or radio daily forecast. Also, look on the EPA's Internet site at <www.epa.gov/sunwise/uvindex.html>.

Stash it everywhere. Never hang your skin out to dry no matter where you are. Keep a bottle of sunscreen in all sorts of places, like your car, pocketbook, picnic basket, or golf bag. And don't worry — leaving sunscreen out in the heat won't affect how it works.

Be a good role model. Teach your children and grandchildren a valuable lesson. Put your sunscreen on in front of them, and they'll follow your lead to healthy skin.

Put men on alert. It's a scientific fact. Men use sunscreen less often than women and are less careful about how they put it on. That means, men, you're more likely to get a sunburn — and more likely to get melanoma after 40. That's a high price to pay for a little carelessness.

Go for the shade. The best way to avoid burning is to stay out of the sun. Find cover under a tree, a beach umbrella, or a wide-brimmed hat. Wear loose-fitting pants and long-sleeved shirts to protect your arms and legs.

Be especially careful from 10 a.m. until 4 p.m. when the sun is strongest. And remember, just because it's cloudy doesn't mean it's safe. About 80 percent of ultraviolet rays can pass through the clouds and cause skin damage.

Skip the reflection. Sand and water can reflect up to 85 percent of the ultraviolet rays. That makes the beach one big magnifying glass, and gives you one more good reason to cover up and slap on sunscreen.

Fake a tan. If you want that attractive summer glow without the risk of cancer, wrinkles, and freckles, experiment with one of the new sunless tanning lotions on the market. These actually stain your skin without harming it. Your "tan" will fade in a week or so, but remember, you'll still need to apply sunscreen.

Nutritious way to clear your mouth of cancer

Each year 30,000 people find out they have mouth or throat cancer, and about 8,000 will die from it. Luckily, you can help avoid this common and deadly cancer by choosing what you put in your mouth.

Eat lots of delicious orange, yellow, and green vegetables and fruits and you could help heal precancerous mouth lesions, and prevent them from developing into cancer. It's the beta carotene (an antioxidant) in these foods that does the trick. One study found that 60 milligrams (mg) of beta carotene a day for six months improved the disease and continued to stay active in the body for several months after the trial.

Check the chart below for examples of foods that will help you get plenty of mouth-healing beta carotene naturally.

Food	Beta carotene
Apricots, 1 cup canned	17 mg
Pumpkin, 1 cup canned	17 mg
Sweet potato, 1 baked	10 mg
Butternut squash, 1 cup cooked	9 mg
Carrots, 1 medium raw	6 mg
Tomato paste, 6 ounces	2 mg

Not sure what a precancerous lesion looks like? Check for white or red patches anywhere in your mouth, or a mouth sore that doesn't heal. Other symptoms of oral cancer include pain or numbness in your mouth or on your lips, a lump in your cheek, jaw swelling, and bad breath.

If you use tobacco products of any kind or drink alcohol, you're more likely to develop oral cancer. If you dip snuff or chew tobacco, your risk increases 50 times! So, spit out that tobacco and chew on some carrots instead.

Brew a pot of protection

Choosing the right beverage could mean less risk of skin cancer.

Green tea contains polyphenols, compounds that act as cancer-fighting antioxidants. These compounds seem to protect skin from the sun's ultraviolet (UV) rays.

Make green tea your drink of choice or apply the extract directly onto your skin. Green tea creams and lotions can reduce the number of sunburn cells and protect your DNA from UV damage.

Experts stress, four or more cups a day may protect against — not cure — cancer. And until there's hard evidence from more research, keep using traditional sunscreen, as well.

TINNITUS

Tame tinnitus with these tactics

Tinnitus and rest don't go together very well. Just try sleeping with a constant ringing, clicking, hissing, roaring, or whistling sound in your ears. That's bad enough, but when you don't get enough rest, your levels of stress and tension increase — and stress and tension can make your tinnitus worse. It's enough to drive you crazy.

What is it?

Tinnitus is a ringing or buzzing sound that only you can hear. Almost any ear disorder, some type of head injury, or certain medications — even aspirin — can cause it. This problem usually goes hand in hand with hearing loss.

Symptoms: ·
- Periodic or constant sounds — ringing, buzzing, hissing, roaring, or whistling
- Hearing loss

"There's no question that stress and tension do exacerbate tinnitus," says Jack Vernon, one of the foremost experts on the condition. "So you want to avoid that if at all possible."

While there's no cure for tinnitus, there are plenty of management strategies. Read on to discover how you can take steps to deal with tinnitus, handle stress, and get the rest you need.

Run a background check. "I tell patients two conditions to religiously avoid," says Vernon, former director of the Oregon Hearing Research Center. "The first is loud sounds because we know they can permanently increase tinnitus. The second is total quiet. Always have some background sound playing."

This approach, called "masking," covers up the sound of the tinnitus, which becomes much more noticeable in complete silence. Masking devices you wear in your ear, like hearing aids, are available. You can also try music; tapes of environmental sounds; or other soothing, distracting noises. The Oregon Hearing Research Center sells Moses-Lang compact discs, which contain seven 10-minute bands of noise, each at an increasingly higher pitch. You can listen to the CD, find the noise that best blocks out your tinnitus, and set your bedside CD player on repeat so you hear that noise all night long. An even simpler solution is to adjust your bedside FM radio between stations so you get static. This often masks tinnitus.

And yet, not everyone responds to masking. "I tell them to do the faucet test," Vernon says. "Go to the kitchen sink and turn the water on full force. If the sound of running water makes it impossible, or nearly so, to hear the tinnitus, it's highly likely that masking will work for them."

The following treatments are similar to masking.

- ↪ **Hearing aids.** Sometimes simply treating your hearing loss helps mask your tinnitus. That's because you suddenly hear the creaks, whirs, and other background sounds of everyday life that you've been missing. These background sounds effectively block out the tinnitus. You can even find a combination hearing aid/masking device if neither one helps by itself.

- ↪ **Tinnitus Retraining Therapy (TRT).** This technique combines low-level, steady background sounds with one-on-one counseling until you grow unaware of tinnitus and eventually no longer need to wear devices in your ears. Although quite effective, TRT can take up to two years to work. "I think most people are interested in more rapid relief," Vernon says.

Attack anxiety. If masking doesn't work, Vernon recommends the anti-anxiety drug Xanax, whose generic name is alprazolam. In a study conducted at Oregon Health Sciences University, 76 percent of those treated with alprazolam experienced relief from tinnitus. The decibel (dB) level of their tinnitus also decreased.

"When loudness was actually measured, it went from a 7.5 dB average to a 2.3 dB average," Vernon says. "If people can get down to 2.3 dB, there will be dancing in the streets."

Of course, Xanax will also help your anxiety and stress. Ask your doctor about this prescription medication. You might also want to try sleep medications if the nighttime is especially difficult for you.

If you'd rather not rely on drugs, try these other stress-busting strategies.

- **Relaxation therapy and visualization.** By using focused breathing and positive imagery, you learn to relax. That means less stress and, possibly, less severe tinnitus.

- **Biofeedback.** This helps you monitor and control your body's reaction to stress. Often used in conjunction with relaxation therapy, biofeedback uses your own nervous system as an ally in the fight to stay healthy.

- **Yoga or meditation.** These methods of relaxation and focusing help some people with tinnitus.

- **Exercise.** Sometimes activity can be distracting. While you're jogging or playing tennis, you're not focusing on the tinnitus.

Join the club. You're not in this alone. Look for a tinnitus support group where you can learn from others and share your experiences with the condition. Many people find this helpful.

It might also be a good idea to join the American Tinnitus Association. This organization sponsors research for tinnitus. The more support it gets, the more research it can sponsor — and the closer they will get to a cure. Plus, becoming a member will help keep you up to date on the latest breakthroughs.

On top of that, feel free to call Vernon for advice. Although he's retired, he still fields telephone calls on Fridays. You can reach him at 503-494-2187. "I'd like to believe we're helping a lot of people with this approach," he says.

Remember, you don't have to use just one treatment option. Mix and match and find what works for you — but do something.

Culprits that threaten your hearing

Limiting your exposure to loud noise helps guard against tinnitus. But noise isn't the only threat to your ears. According to the American Tinnitus Association, the following common items can make your tinnitus worse.

- Certain medications
- Caffeine
- Alcohol
- Nicotine
- High-sugar foods
- Tonic water
- Stress
- Fatigue

Now that you know the possible culprits, you can take steps to protect yourself.

Let your doctor know what medications — both prescription and over-the-counter drugs — you're taking. Cut out nicotine, which affects your hearing by constricting the blood vessels carrying oxygen to your ears. Limit caffeine and alcohol and any other foods that seem to make your tinnitus worse. And try to relax.

Not everyone reacts the same way to these items, so you don't have to give up everything. Find out what makes the ringing in your ears worse and adjust your lifestyle accordingly.

Now hear this: Vacuuming can harm ears

Explosions and machinegun fire can put a soldier's hearing as well as his life at risk. But you don't have to be a veteran of the battlefield to suffer noise-induced hearing loss. Many objects in your own home can also damage your ears — vacuum cleaners, garbage disposals, leaf blowers, and shop tools.

Sound is measured in units called decibels. To get an idea of how loud a decibel is, normal conversation is about 60 decibels. Any sound above 75 decibels has the potential to cause hearing loss. A sudden loud noise, like an explosion, or loud noises over a long period of time, like continuous sounds in your workplace, can damage the delicate hair cells or hearing nerves in your ears. This can lead to hearing loss or tinnitus.

According to the American Tinnitus Association, everyday noises that might cause hearing loss include:

- Blow dryer — 100 decibels
- Subway — 100 decibels
- Power lawn mower — 105 decibels
- Chainsaw — 105 decibels
- Motorcycle — 120 decibels
- Fireworks — 120 decibels
- Shotgun blast — 140 decibels

Recreational activities like woodworking, riding snowmobiles or go-carts, target shooting, and hunting also endanger your ears. In fact, a recent University of Wisconsin study found that men who regularly engage in target shooting are 57 percent more likely to have hearing loss than those who don't. And the more years you hunt, the greater your risk of hearing loss. To make matters worse, a third of the target shooters and almost all of the hunters reported never wearing hearing protection.

Even if you don't use firearms, noise can mean big trouble for your ears. More than 30 million people are exposed to high-decibel sounds on a regular basis, whether at work, at play, or at home. Here's how to protect yourself.

Know your enemy. Be aware of what noises might harm your ears. Make sure your family, friends, co-workers, and especially children are protected against noises louder than 75 decibels.

Block your ears. Wear earplugs or earmuffs when you participate in a loud activity. These can prevent both kinds of hearing loss — that caused by a brief impulse (explosion) or the kind caused by continuous exposure. You can find them at hardware or sporting goods stores.

Get a check-up. Sometimes hearing loss is so gradual you might not notice it until it's too late. Schedule an examination by an ear, nose, and throat specialist and a hearing test by an audiologist, a health professional who can detect and measure hearing loss.

Taking these precautions will make your day-to-day encounters with noise a little easier on your ears. And remember, before you plug in that vacuum cleaner, put in some earplugs.

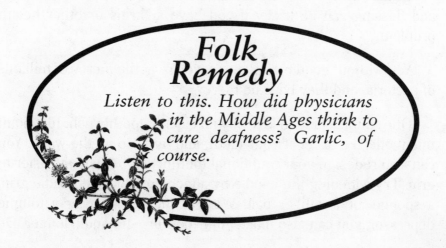

Folk
Remedy

Listen to this. How did physicians in the Middle Ages think to cure deafness? Garlic, of course.

TOOTHACHE

Preventing cavities in 'grown-up' teeth

Less than one out of three seniors has dentures today. Only 30 years ago, more than two out of three seniors had false teeth. These statistics sound like a dental miracle, but if you're a senior with your natural teeth, think about this. More than 95 percent of seniors have receding gum lines, and this leaves their roots open to attack by decay-causing bacteria. No wonder tooth decay is three times as likely in seniors as it is in children.

How can this be? Teeth you've had your entire lifetime can wear out just like any other part of your body. There are also other reasons why your teeth are under attack, and all of them are under your control.

Brush like you were 20 again. Doing a good job brushing and flossing can be tricky if you have arthritis or other health problems.

Yet, without good oral hygiene, you're at the mercy of millions of bacteria, and they have no mercy.

One simple solution is to buy an electric toothbrush. Just point this modern marvel at your teeth, and let it do all the work. You can also redesign your traditional toothbrush to make it easier to grip. Try widening the handle by attaching a bicycle handle grip, a sponge, or a rubber ball. With a wooden ruler or a tongue depressor, you can also make your toothbrush handle longer. Do both by wrapping adhesive tape around your toothbrush until the handle is the perfect length and width. For flossing ease, make your string into a loop or buy a special floss holder.

Ask your doctor about side effects. Medications that cause dry mouth could be putting you at risk for tooth decay. These include decongestants, antihistamines, painkillers, and diuretics. Saliva not only lubricates your mouth, it washes away food that normally gets stuck between your teeth. More importantly, it diluates the bacterial acid that causes cavities. That's why a parched mouth spells trouble for your teeth.

To get your juices flowing again, talk with your doctor about switching medications. In some cases, she might be able to prescribe another medicine that won't sap your saliva. For quick relief, enjoy a piece of sugar-free candy or gum. They encourage your salivary glands to produce more saliva.

Don't turn your back on fluoride. Drinking bottled or purified water might be putting your mouth in danger. That's because these sources of water are short on fluoride, the mineral that's famous for guarding teeth. Most towns and cities add fluoride to their water supplies, but if you're drinking bottled or purified water, you're missing out.

What is it?

The pain you experience in or around a tooth may come from one easily identified spot. You might feel an ache when you chew or bite down, or when you eat or drink something hot, cold, or sweet. This could mean the protective layer on your tooth has decayed, exposing the sensitive nerves. A simple filling should fix this problem.

However, your discomfort could also come from a tooth abscess, gum disease, impacted wisdom teeth, or inflamed sinuses.

Symptoms:
- Dull or sharp tooth pain
- Tender or swollen gums
- Swelling of the face and neck
- Fever

If you don't want to give up your bottled water, consider this surprising source of fluoride — carbonated soft drinks. Most brands, according to recent research, contain almost as much fluoride as most tap water. But remember, the sugar could undo any benefit the fluoride has. If you enjoy an occasional soft drink, stick with the sugar-free varieties.

Leave your fears behind. Avoiding the dentist can be downright dangerous, leading to tooth loss and gum disease.

Dentistry has come a long way. Gone are the days of painful drilling with a foot-pedaled drill. Dentists today have the talent and the technology to make your next visit comfortably pain-free. If you're unhappy with your dentist, find one that helps you feel comfortable. Don't let bad memories from your childhood prevent you from having a healthy mouth.

Snack wisely. Experts say when you eat is as important as what you eat. Eating during scheduled meal times is much better for your teeth than nibbling on snacks throughout the day. Each snack you eat leaves your teeth open to attack from bacteria for at least 20 minutes. Meals cause less damage because you have more saliva in your mouth during a full meal. If you have to snack, stick with these nutritious choices — veggies, cheese, plain yogurt, or a piece of fruit.

Listen up, denture wearers. Don't think you can avoid taking care of your mouth just because you wear dentures. According to experts, you're still at risk for mouth cancer, gum disease, and mouth sores.

Visit your dentist at least once a year. She can check your mouth for signs of trouble and make sure your dentures fit well.

Natural weapons wipe out decay

A war is going on in your mouth, and your teeth are outnumbered a million to one. Armies of bacteria are swarming, growing into sticky clumps called plaque, and setting up strongholds in your mouth. Once they attach themselves to your teeth, they'll feast on the sugar in your mouth and leave behind an acid that can cause cavities, abscesses, and gum disease.

Daily brushing and flossing is the best strategy to even the odds in this war. To finish off your enemy, send in the reserves — natural remedies to help keep your teeth strong.

Wash away decay with wasabi. It's already famous for preventing cancer, heart disease, and asthma, but now this green-colored Japanese horseradish is making a name for itself fighting

When is a toothache not a toothache?

You might not need to open your mouth for that next root canal. According to dental experts, the following conditions — not tooth decay — could be causing your "toothache."

- **Sinus infection.** If you feel pain bending over, suffer from chronic allergies, had a recent cold, or just flew on a plane, your ache could signal an infection called acute maxillary sinusitis (AMS). Instead of a root canal, all you need are the right prescription medicines.
- **Neurological disorder.** Nerve problems — like Atypical Facial Pain (AFP) and Trigeminal Neuralgia — might be causing your discomfort. Your dentist can recommend a good neurologist.
- **Cancer.** Tingling or numbness could also signal a much more serious problem — oral cancer. Though it's rare, play it safe and let your dentist have a look.
- **Bruxism.** Grinding your teeth can become a painful habit. Talk with your dentist about how to kick it.

To stop the pain of these conditions, make sure you get a proper diagnosis. Otherwise, you might be in for some unnecessary drilling — and that's a jaw-dropping thought.

tooth decay. According to a recent study, chemicals in wasabi called isothiocyanates stop bacteria from sticking to your teeth. Try the spicy condiment the next time you're at a sushi restaurant. Better yet, stockpile some at home and experiment with it in your own dishes. Just remember — a little of this fiery topping goes a long way.

Enjoy a cup of tea. If you want to declare a D-Day on those bacteria in your mouth, learn a lesson from the British and take time for tea. Black tea, the most popular beverage in the world after water, appears to be one of the biggest enemies of cavity-causing bacteria. It kills some of them in their tracks and flushes out the rest before they stick to your teeth. Green tea seems to battle tooth decay, too. Whichever type of tea you prefer, remember to drink it plain. Adding milk or sugar will just give the bacteria the ammo they need to fight back.

Sweeten your smile. Honey is so good at killing bacteria and healing infections that doctors around the world use it to treat burns, ulcers, and now tooth decay. Experts believe honey works by releasing hydrogen peroxide, a chemical that's not so sweet for bacteria. Not all types of honey have this power. Unprocessed kinds, like you'd find at a health food store, pack the best hydrogen peroxide punch.

Brush with chocolate. Chocolate toothpaste and mouthwash could be the wave of the future if recent research holds true. Scientists in Japan have found chemicals in cocoa bean husks that can stop cavity-causing bacteria from growing and sticking to your teeth. This doesn't mean you should feast on a candy bar before bed. The sugar would outweigh the benefits of the antibacterial chemicals. Instead, it's best to wait for the chocolate toothpastes of the future.

Shy away from germs. Pucker up with the wrong person, and you could catch a cavity. Experts say cavity-causing bacteria can hitch a ride from mouth to mouth. Also, be careful about sharing other people's eating utensils. Bacteria can be passed from a spoon, fork, or sipping straw.

It's important to remember that these remedies can't replace brushing and flossing. When you use them along with good oral hygiene, however, these natural remedies can help you win the war against tooth decay.

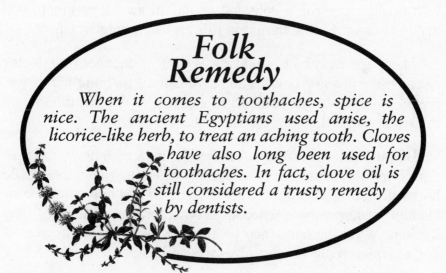

Folk
Remedy

When it comes to toothaches, spice is nice. The ancient Egyptians used anise, the licorice-like herb, to treat an aching tooth. Cloves have also long been used for toothaches. In fact, clove oil is still considered a trusty remedy by dentists.

URINARY INCONTINENCE

Don't let laughter dampen your mood

When you were younger, the idea of laughing until you wet your pants may have been a joke. However, if you have problems with bladder control, a common condition in older women, you may no longer see the humor in this embarrassing situation.

There are many causes and cures of incontinence. Your doctor can advise you about devices and medications that might help you regain control of your bladder. In addition, there are things you can try at home that may do the trick.

Boost your hormones. Although younger women may experience urinary incontinence, especially when pregnant, the female hormone estrogen generally keeps the muscles that control your bladder strong. After menopause, however, these muscles may weaken. When incontinence is hormone related, some women find estrogen replacement solves the problem.

Give your drugs a double take. Another cause of incontinence could be lurking in your medicine cabinet — in high blood pressure capsules, cold formulas, water pills, or other medications.

Stopping or changing to another medication may be the answer for you, but never quit taking a prescription without first discussing it with your doctor.

Exercise some control. Pregnancy and childbirth affect your life and your body in many ways. Unfortunately, weakened pelvic muscles often come with the territory. Women who've had several children seem to especially suffer from incontinence later in life.

Kegels are exercises that can strengthen the muscles that help you hold urine in your bladder. Try squeezing the muscles you use to stop urinating. Hold them tight for about 10 seconds, and then relax for the same amount of time. Do this 10 times a day.

Don't tighten leg, stomach, or other muscles. This can put more pressure on the muscles that control your bladder. If you aren't sure you're exercising the right muscles, ask your doctor or nurse about it.

Gradually increase the number of times you do the exercises until you are completing at least three sets of 10 each day. To really strengthen these muscles, use three different positions — lying, sitting, and standing.

Be patient. This requires practice, as with any muscle-building plan. It may take weeks to see results, but doing Kegels regularly will pay off. Most of the women who do them correctly — and keep doing them — can see results even 10 years later.

Retrain your bladder. Certain medical conditions can affect bladder control. If you've had nerve damage from diabetes or a stroke, if you suffer from some type of infection, or if you have trouble walking because of an illness, you may need to use particular strategies to help restore your former bladder habits.

> ### *What is it?*
>
> If you have trouble holding or controlling your urine, there's usually a problem with the muscles in your bladder or surrounding your urethra. It is not just a symptom of aging and is often temporary.
>
> Stress incontinence, the most common kind, is likely to occur when laughing, coughing, sneezing, or exercising puts pressure on the bladder causing urine to leak out. Pregnancy, menopause, and the structure of the female anatomy mean this is more common in women than in men.
>
> Symptoms:
> - Leaking urine
> - Incomplete emptying of the bladder, leading to overflow

Eat, drink, and don't leak

Don't drink less water in the hopes of stemming a leaky bladder. Your body needs water — at least six glasses a day. However, certain other beverages and foods might affect incontinence. Experiment by eliminating these items from your diet one at a time for seven to 10 days.

- Caffeinated beverages such as coffee and tea
- Carbonated beverages
- Citrus fruits
- Tomatoes and tomato-based foods
- Spicy foods
- Chocolate
- Sugar and honey
- Milk and milk products

Your doctor may suggest, for example, that you go to the bathroom at specific intervals, perhaps every hour. If you stay dry for the hour, she may recommend increasing the intervals to an hour and a half.

Follow these tips and soon you'll be ready to enjoy jokes again. Just remember to tighten those pelvic muscles before you laugh, and do the same before you sneeze, lift, or jump. You'll have fewer accidents, and you'll help protect your muscles from more damage.

Speak up to stay dry

If you can just get over the embarrassment and talk to your doctor, you can probably get help for your bladder problems. Remember, this is an issue for millions of women and you don't have to face it alone.

First, ask your doctor if he handles bladder problems. If not, get a recommendation for one who does. Then, organize your thoughts in advance. This way you'll be more confident when it's time to discuss the details of this personal issue.

Go armed with answers. Your doctor will probably ask about your current and past illnesses, accidents, and surgeries. He may want to know if you have reached menopause. If you've given birth, he may ask about your deliveries. Expect questions about your diet and any medications, both prescription and over-the-counter, you take.

Be ready to report when your incontinence began, how often it occurs, and what you experience — burning or pain, for instance.

Plan your own questions. Ask if it would help to make changes in what you eat or drink. Find out if one or more of your medicines could be causing the problem and if another medication would work just as well without this side effect. Inquire about exercises and bladder retraining programs.

Finding the cause of your incontinence requires clear communication and is the only way to determine what treatment is best for you.

Stop incontinence from tripping you up

That sudden, overpowering need to go to the bathroom can rule your days — and your nights. This problem, called urge incontinence, spells trouble two ways.

Heed the risk to men. While more common in women, urge incontinence may be a more significant health issue in men. If you are a man who has this happen at night, especially if it doesn't occur in the daytime, see your doctor right away. You could have a severe blockage of your prostate or bladder. It could also mean you're suffering from a serious complication in your urinary tract.

Sidestep nighttime dangers. "Women who have urge incontinence get up often to urinate at night — jumping out of the bed and rushing to the bathroom to prevent urine leakage," says Dr. Jeanette S. Brown, a specialist in women's incontinence at the University of California, San Francisco.

In your mad dash for the bathroom, you are likely to trip and fall. In fact, urge incontinence increases your risk of falling by 26 percent. And falling means fractures — a major health concern for older women, in particular.

"We are looking for simple ways," says Brown, "to prevent falls and fractures and keep women active." She recommends treatments that don't require surgery, such as bladder retraining or medications. Talk to your doctor about these possibilities.

Injuries caused by incontinence happen in the daytime, too. So, protect yourself from bumps and breaks by clearing a safe pathway to the toilet. And perhaps, as Brown suggests, get a bedside commode for nighttime emergencies.

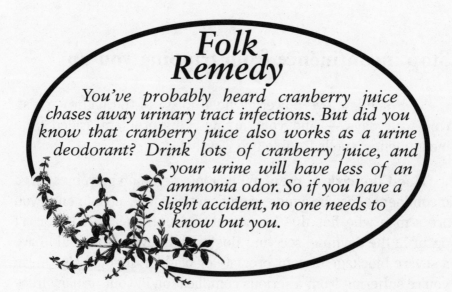

Folk Remedy

You've probably heard cranberry juice chases away urinary tract infections. But did you know that cranberry juice also works as a urine deodorant? Drink lots of cranberry juice, and your urine will have less of an ammonia odor. So if you have a slight accident, no one needs to know but you.

VARICOSE VEINS

Vanquish varicose veins naturally

Varicose veins are achy, painful, and even dangerous because of possible blood clots. But they're also ugly. The blue, swollen tangle of veins can transform your once fetching legs into unsightly road maps.

If you want to keep your legs looking good without resorting to surgery, follow these helpful guidelines.

- ❧ **Change your diet.** Load up on fiber and cut down on saturated fat, salt, and processed foods. Eat plenty of fruits, vegetables, and whole grains. This will help head off constipation, which contributes to varicose veins. In addition to fiber, fruits and vegetables also provide vitamins C and E, which help strengthen your circulatory system.

- ❧ **Exercise.** Come up with a regular, moderate exercise routine. Walking, swimming, and yoga give your leg muscles a good workout, but be careful not to overdo it. "If someone has varicose veins and

> ### *What is it?*
>
> You have valves in your veins that keep the blood flowing properly. When they become defective, the blood pools, making the veins swell and twist. These are called varicose veins and they're most common in your legs.
>
> Women are more prone to varicose veins than men. Obesity, pregnancy, and standing for a long time can contribute to the problem.
>
> Symptoms:
> - ❧ Blue, swollen, twisted veins
> - ❧ Aching, made worse by prolonged standing
> - ❧ Swollen feet and ankles
> - ❧ Itching

is killing themselves marathon running or becoming dehydrated, they're not doing any good," says George Nemecz, a biochemistry professor at Campbell University in North Carolina.

↪ **Lose weight.** A combination of a healthy diet and a solid exercise program should help you shed those extra pounds, which pose an extra risk for varicose veins.

↪ **Wear comfortable clothing.** Tight clothes, especially garments that fit too snugly around your waist, can obstruct circulation. So can high heels. Opt for loose clothing and flats instead.

↪ **Don't stand still.** If you need to be on your feet for long stretches of time, rock from one leg to the other or pace back and forth to keep your muscles moving.

↪ **Slip on support hose.** These elastic stockings offer relief from your calves to your thighs. They come in handy if you must stand a lot for your job, if you're pregnant, or if you're overweight. Custom-made compression stockings can help in more severe cases. Put either type of stocking on early in the morning, before the blood gets a chance to pool in your lower legs.

↪ **Modify your bed.** Raising the foot of your bed by about six inches helps keep the pressure off your veins at night. With your legs elevated, the blood should flow away from your aching calves. You can use wooden blocks or books to raise the foot of your bed.

↪ **Don't cross your legs.** This cuts off circulation. Instead, when you sit down, use a footstool to keep your feet level with, or even slightly higher than, your hips.

↪ **Soak in hot and cold.** Alternating between cold and hot water constricts and dilates your blood vessels.

Your vessels get a workout and become stronger. Nemecz suggests keeping your legs in cold water for about 15 minutes and then switching to warm water for several minutes.

- **Stop smoking.** This unhealthy habit narrows your blood vessels so blood has trouble moving through your body.

- **Know your family history.** Thin skin, weak veins, and poor circulation might run in your family. If your mother

---

'Plane' and simple travel tips

A 28-year-old woman died recently from a blood clot after flying from Australia to London. Her death brought attention to "economy-class syndrome," which refers to the cramped conditions of airlines' coach seating.

But the real problem is sitting still for long periods of time — even if you fly first class. In fact, riding in buses or cars, or even just sitting at your desk, for extended periods can be just as dangerous as flying.

If you have varicose veins, you're at even greater risk of developing a potentially deadly blood clot. Here are some tips for traveling safely.

- Wear compression stockings, which drastically reduced the risk of blood clots on long flights in a recent study.
- Move your legs and feet. On a plane, get up and walk around the cabin every hour. If you're driving, stop every couple of hours to walk around.
- Exercise your calf muscles while sitting.
- Ask your doctor if he recommends taking a low-dose aspirin before flying.
- Drink plenty of water, but avoid alcohol and beverages with caffeine.
- Wear loose-fitting clothing.
- Don't cross your legs.
- Know the risk factors, including obesity, pregnancy, and family history, and talk with your doctor if you're concerned.

---

had varicose veins, you should take precautions so you don't develop the condition, too.

Fortify your veins with herbs

Surgery and drugs can clear up varicose veins, but why not try something gentler, like herbs? Plants, after all, are the root of all medicine and the foundation of good health. But don't think you can just pop a few herbs and expect a magical recovery. You still need to stick to a sensible diet, exercise regularly, and maintain a healthy weight.

Also, make sure to follow your doctor's advice. For example, if he recommends compression stockings, wear them — and let him know you're thinking of taking herbs.

Which herbs help varicose veins?

"Any herbs that have antioxidants and also help with microcirculation — hawthorn, grape seed extract, yarrow, and ginkgo," says George Nemecz, a biochemistry professor at Campbell University in North Carolina. Microcirculation refers to blood flow in the very small blood vessels.

Following are some herbs that help improve circulation and soothe the symptoms of varicose veins.

Horse chestnut seed extract. Perhaps the most effective herbal remedy for varicose veins, horse chestnut seed extract reduces inflammation, improves blood flow, and strengthens your veins. A review by University of Exeter researchers showed that horse chestnut seed extract worked better than a placebo and just as well as some medications to ease the symptoms of varicose veins. Its secret is a substance called escin. According to German experts, you should aim for 100 milligrams (mg) of ecsin a day. This means taking a daily dosage of horse chestnut seed extract that ranges from 250 to 312.5 mg twice a day.

Ginkgo biloba. This multipurpose herb does wonders for blood flow, especially in the tiny capillaries that connect arteries to veins. It also protects the walls of your blood vessels and strengthens your capillaries. Ginkgo won't heal varicose veins, but it will help prevent you from developing more. Take 120 to 160 mg two or three times a day.

Butcher's broom. Sweep away the pain, heaviness, and swelling of varicose veins with Butcher's broom. This ancient herb reduces inflammation and firms up your veins. In one study, scientists found that symptoms of varicose veins, including itching, tingling, and cramping, improved when subjects took a drug that included extracts of this herb. The two main active ingredients are ruscogenin and neoruscogenin. You should get 7 to 11 mg of total ruscogenin (ruscogenin plus neoruscogenin) each day.

Gotu kola. This ancient Ayurvedic herb — used for a wide range of problems, including depression, high blood pressure, and wounds — improves blood flow while strengthening veins and capillaries. One study showed an extract of this plant helped varicose veins more than a placebo.

"The mechanism is not quite clear," Nemecz says of the reason for gotu kola's positive effect on blood vessels. But he adds, "The formation of clots and pressure on the wall and elasticity of the wall is better in the presence of gotu kola."

Nemecz says a number of ingredients, including asiatic acid, may be responsible. A typical daily dose is 600 mg of dried leaves. You can also take capsules, which range from 300 mg to 680 mg, three times a day.

Garlic. This fragrant bulb helps keep your blood from clumping or becoming too sticky. This keeps your blood moving through your blood vessels and reduces the risk of blood clots. One clove a day — about 4 grams of fresh garlic — should do the trick. You can also take garlic capsules.

Get to the bottom of hemorrhoids

Not all swollen veins are found in your legs. Often, they show up as hemorrhoids. These painful, itching masses form inside your rectum or on the surface of your anus.

What's more, they can bleed. Report any bleeding to your doctor because it could indicate a more serious condition — like colon cancer.

In most cases, you can fight hemorrhoids on your own with these self-help tips.

- Eat a high-fiber diet. This means more fruits, vegetables, and whole grains.
- Drink plenty of water. Along with fiber, this helps keep stools soft and easy to pass.
- Change your bathroom habits. Straining contributes to hemorrhoids, but just sitting on the toilet too long may be the main culprit.
- Soak in warm baths that cover only your hips and buttocks.
- Exercise regularly.
- Seek over-the-counter help. Look for products with benzo-caine, dibucaine, pramoxine, or hydrocortisone to relieve burning and itching. You can also use witch hazel, petroleum jelly, cocoa butter, or mineral oil.
- Try herbal remedies. Herbs that might help include Butcher's broom, horse chestnut, Gotu kola, St. John's wort, and flaxseed.

Grape seed extract. Powerful antioxidant compounds make grape seed extract a mighty weapon against varicose veins. Called pycnogenols, these compounds are also found in pine bark extract. Like garlic, they improve blood flow and stop your blood from clumping and clotting. Herbal experts recommend taking 50 mg a day.

Witch hazel. This remedy, also good for hemorrhoids, involves applying the extract to your skin. You can find witch hazel in stores, but because of a process called steam distilling, most of the tannins — the substances that help shrink swollen veins — have been removed. For more effective witch hazel, look for nondistilled hydroalcoholic extracts, which might be difficult to find. Or you can boil 5 to 10 heaping teaspoons of finely chopped witch hazel leaves in a cup of water for five to 10 minutes, then strain and use as a poultice.

Hawthorn. Although recommended mostly for heart problems, hawthorn leaf and flower preparations can also help with blood flow in your legs. The various flavonoids in hawthorn give the herb its power. To make an herbal tea, add a handful of fresh or dried hawthorn flowers to boiled water and steep for about 15 minutes. Herbalists recommend drinking one to three cups a day.

Yarrow. Like witch hazel, yarrow is an astringent that fights inflammation and cramps. Soak in a sitz bath — only up to your belly button — that consists of 100 grams (3.5 ounces) of yarrow for every 5 gallons of water.

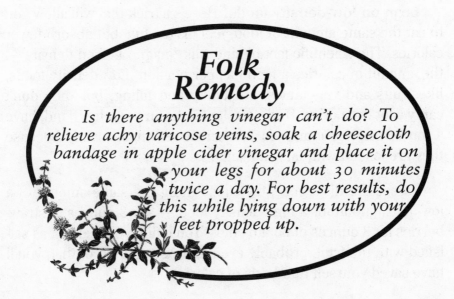

Folk Remedy

Is there anything vinegar can't do? To relieve achy varicose veins, soak a cheesecloth bandage in apple cider vinegar and place it on your legs for about 30 minutes twice a day. For best results, do this while lying down with your feet propped up.

WEIGHT PROBLEMS

Trick your body into losing weight

Do you turn to tricks and traps to lose weight? Weight-loss pills may sound like the answer to prayers, but these drugs can do more harm than good, not to mention costing you an arm and a leg. And single-food diets promising miracles can be nutritional nightmares. What you need are some healthy tricks that will melt those pounds off naturally and easily.

Lean on low-density foods. Here's a trick that will allow you to eat the same amount of food, feel just as full, but absorb fewer calories. The scientific fact behind this "magic" is food density — the amount of calories a food has per portion. Low-density foods, like fruits and vegetables, are bulky and filling, but they don't carry a lot of calories. High-density foods, on the other hand, have a ton of calories crammed into small servings, mainly because they are loaded with fats and sugars.

To see the difference, try substituting the same amount of a low-density food for a high-density food — say 3 ounces of strawberries for 3 ounces of potato chips. You'll find you feel just as satisfied with the fruit, probably even more so. On top of that, you'll have saved yourself hundreds of calories.

Your goal is to eat more low-density foods such as produce, whole grains, and legumes, and cut down on fatty, sugary foods. But remember — even low-fat or fat-free snacks can be high-density because of their tremendous sugar content.

Fluff up your food. You may remember adding fluff to your peanut butter sandwiches as a child. That sugary confection will not help you lose weight, but food with extra air whipped in just might. A study at Pennsylvania State University found these "fluffy" foods could help you eat less.

In the study, 28 men drank one of three different kinds of milkshakes before lunch. All three milkshakes had the same ingredients, but some were blended longer to add air and volume. The men who drank the "airy" shakes ate 12 percent fewer calories at lunch.

> ### What is it?
> Your healthiest weight is determined by considering your height-to-weight ratio or Body Mass Index (BMI), and the amount and location of body fat. Being either overweight or underweight can lead to health problems.
>
> Symptoms:
> - A BMI greater than 25
> - Weight that exceeds or falls below the ideal as shown in weight-for-height tables
> - Waistline measurements of more than 35 inches for women and 40 inches for men

And they did not make up for it by eating more at dinner, meaning they kept those calories off.

So if you must snack, trick your senses by filling up on an air-filled treat like low-fat frozen yogurt or butter-free popcorn.

Shrink your serving sizes. Cleaning your plate could be one of the only bad habits your mom taught you. Especially if you eat at a typical restaurant with a mountain of food on your platter. According to a recent study, the more you have on your plate, the more you'll eat. Fortunately, the opposite is true as well.

One great way to limit your serving size is to cook at home, where you can control how much food you cook. You also can try eating off a smaller plate to reduce the size of your portions.

Things get trickier when you eat out, but there are ways around a restaurant's generosity. Overcome huge entrées by splitting them with your spouse or friend. If you go it alone, put half your dinner into a doggie bag before you even start eating. That way, you won't be tempted by a full plate.

Limit food variety. A wide selection of food may be appealing when you're at a buffet, but it won't be when you get on the scale afterward. An overload of food appears to make your stomach's fuel gauge shut down. You're more likely to go beyond "full" just so you can taste everything. Experts think this tendency comes from our ancestors, who had to eat a variety of foods to guarantee they got all their nutrients.

The trick is to limit your snack selection. Store only one brand of chips in your cupboard or one type of cake in your fridge. You'll end up snacking less often because you'll get tired of the same old taste. On the other hand, stockpile a wide selection of fruits and vegetables. Variety in this case means getting a mix of nutrients and phytochemicals that would make your ancestors envious.

Ditch high-calorie drinks. You've heard of a beer belly, but how about a soda belly? Experts say you can put on pounds without realizing it by drinking high-calorie beverages. Your body doesn't seem to register the drinks because they go right through you. So you take in hundreds of empty calories, and your stomach is still hungry for more.

Do yourself a favor, and replace most of your high-calorie drinks with low- or no-calorie ones like tea and water. You'll quench your thirst and save some pounds.

7 ways fiber helps you win at losing

You've tried the hot dog diet, the banana diet, and the grapefruit diet. You've gone through diet pills, sweat suits, and supplements.

Don't be fooled by food labels

Food labels provide useful information if you're trying to improve your eating habits. In fact, a recent study found that reading food labels helps you trim the fat from your diet. But don't believe everything you read. A *Consumer Reports* feature recently pointed out a few labeling loopholes.

- **Hidden fiber content.** If a breakfast cereal has no fiber, the manufacturer can include the phrase "Not a significant source of dietary fiber" below the rest of the nutrient information in smaller type. That way, you might not notice it.
- **Fat-free fibs.** A food can claim to be "fat-free" if it has less than half a gram of fat per serving. That's why pretzels, which actually contain 1 or 2 grams of fat per cup, are considered a fat-free food.
- **Fuzzy math.** Nutrient analyses can be off by as much as 20 percent. This allows for natural variations in food. But it also allows for some confusion. For example, a food that claims to have 200 calories can actually contain anywhere from 160 to 240 calories.

It's a good idea to read labels to help keep track of what you eat. Just remember that what you see is not always what you get.

Your home is littered with exercise equipment and videos that promised to help you lose those extra pounds. But despite your best efforts, you can't seem to lose weight. What are you doing wrong?

Chances are, you're not eating enough fiber. Studies show obesity rates are tied to the amount of fiber people eat. In places like Kenya and Uganda, where they eat as much as 60 to 80 grams of fiber daily, less than 15 percent of the population are overweight. But the measly 15 grams a day eaten in more modern societies like the United States have contributed to the obesity of nearly 60 percent of adults.

If you're one of them, you'll need to change your diet to include more fruits and vegetables because most fiber comes from plants. You'll find it in whole-grain foods, legumes, leafy veg-etables, fruits, nuts, root vegetables and their skins, and bran flakes. Besides allowing you more food on your plate, this impor-tant diet aid works on several levels to keep you trim.

Offers more food per calorie. One of the best things about fiber is that some of its calories don't count. That's because much of dietary fiber can't be digested. But fiber still fills you up. Experts say eating a diet high in fiber can trick your stomach into feeling full with fewer calories than you would normally eat.

Prolongs your meal. Most people would agree that the plea-sure of food lies in the eating. A high-fiber diet requires lots of chewing and swallowing, and it can take a good while to finish a meal. Unlike many diets that limit food, you won't have to give up the joy of eating when you add fiber to your diet. It might actually take you longer than usual to polish off a lower-calorie meal.

Bulks up in your stomach. Ever finish a small meal while dieting and still feel hunger pangs? That won't happen if you eat more fiber. Water-soluble fiber absorbs water from your stomach and forms a kind of gel that swells up. Nerve receptors in your stomach signal your brain that your stomach is full, and you no longer need to eat. By filling up on fiber, you can go about your business without constantly feeling hungry.

Keeps you satisfied longer. But that's not all fiber can do. The thick gel it forms slows down the movement of food out of your stomach, so you end up processing your food more slowly. Instead of a high-calorie blast of energy that is quickly followed by tiredness and hunger, your energy supply is spread out over time.

Stabilizes blood sugar. Experts say this process affects your blood sugar in a healthy way. When you eat dried beans, barley, whole wheat, or pumpernickel bread, these foods slowly release their sugars for energy. Instead of your body getting surges of sugar from food, it gets its energy in steady amounts, which helps control insulin levels. In addition, a high-fiber meal can affect your blood sugar's response to the next meal you eat, keeping your blood sugar more stable throughout the day.

Boosts your hormones. You may not know it, but you have hormones working in your gastrointestinal tract. One in particular, called GLP-1, slows down the digestion process and gives you a sense of fullness. It can also help you lose weight. Studies on animals showed that eating fermentable fiber — the kind in fruits and vegetables — boosted their levels of GLP-1.

Blocks some calories. Dietary fiber can block the absorption of some of the fat and protein you eat. If you're overweight, that could be a good thing. One study showed that a group of people fed a diet containing only 20 grams of fiber a day absorbed 8 percent more calories than a group given 48 grams of fiber a day. For a typical 2,500-calorie diet, that's a difference of about 200 calories a day.

Just changing your fiber intake — without altering the number of calories you eat — could mean losing a couple of pounds a month. But be careful to add fiber to your diet slowly. Too much too soon can cause uncomfortable gas and bloating.

Fitness: The key to good health

Here's some good news if you're over age 65. Losing a lot of pounds and exercising like an Olympian may not be necessary to stay healthy. Instead, all you need are a sensible, steady weight and moderate everyday activity. So take heart if you're on the upper end of the scale — by staying fit, you can help avoid the diseases of old age and still enjoy your golden years.

Disregard the BMI. Experts claim a healthy body mass index (BMI) ranges from 19 to 25. This measure reflects your weight in relation to your height and is calculated by multiplying your weight by 703, then dividing that number by your height in inches squared. Anything above 25 means you're overweight, and above 30, obese.

But lucky for you, scientists found these strict standards don't apply to adults over age 65. After looking at 13 studies on BMI and death rates, they discovered the risk of dying from heart disease and other causes does not go up with a BMI between 25 and 27. It's not until you cross that line that you have to be concerned. A BMI of 28 or above seems to increase your risk of death at any age.

That means it's fine to have a few extra pounds on you as you age. Since you've made it this far with them, your body can obviously handle the extra weight. Having a "nutritional reserve" may even help protect you from some conditions, such as osteoporosis.

Aim to keep fit. The important thing for your health is to stay in shape. According to surprising new research, obese people who are physically fit are less likely to die prematurely than skinny layabouts. That leads experts to believe fitness could be the key to good health — not weight loss. So look at exercise as a way you can stay healthy, not just a way to drop pounds. It's the only health care accessible to everyone — no prescription needed.

Shoot for the recommended 30 minutes of exercise almost every day of the week, but don't feel you need to do it in one lump sum. You can split up the 30 minutes, and spread exercise moments throughout your free time. And don't give up because you think you have no time for the gym, or tennis, or other typical exercises. Raking the leaves, cleaning up around the house, or gardening for 30 minutes counts, too, as does any activity that gets you perspiring and a little out of breath.

Stay moderately active. Moderate exercise is better for you than short bursts of heavy-duty activity, according to a recent study from Europe. In other words, 10 minutes of fast-paced running won't make up for 10 hours spent in front of the boob tube.

But being moderately active all day long — instead of sitting in front of the television — can make a difference.

Living a couch potato's life, experts say, puts you at greater risk for a string of diseases, including arthritis, Type 2 diabetes, obesity, cancer, heart disease, and depression. According to some estimates, inactivity causes the deaths of 250,000 people a year in the United States alone. Experts have coined a new name for this condition marked by chronic inactivity — Sedentary Death Syndrome (SeDS). If you want to avoid SeDS, make it a point to stay active.

Add steps to your day. One way to turn your whole day into a workout is to take 10,000 steps. You probably do a lot of walking already without even thinking about it. The average adult takes 3,000 to 5,000 steps each day. If you punch that number up to 10,000, experts say, you'll get the equivalent of a steady 30-minute workout. Fitness experts in Japan first tried out the idea, and now it has caught on in America. Researchers at Stanford University and at the Cooper Institute in Dallas have researched it and agree that it seems to work.

You can reach 10,000 steps by literally counting every step you take. Rebecca Lindbergh of Health Partners, a managed care organization in Minnesota, coordinates a program in which people actually wear a pedometer to tally their walking. "We encourage them to wear the pedometer all day long," she says about her participants. "They use the pedometer and slip activity in throughout their day." For example, you can:

- Park farther away at the mall.

- Take the steps instead of the escalator or elevator.

- Walk the golf course instead of taking a cart.

- Spend your coffee break on a walk instead of standing around the water cooler.

↜ March through your local mall, and browse every store that catches your fancy.

↜ Walk while you're on the phone or during television commercial breaks.

With a pedometer, you begin to notice how these little changes add up to more and more steps. "Using a pedometer puts a little pizazz into walking," Lindbergh notes. "It's very eye-opening." If you would like to count 10,000 steps, you can find a pedometer at any sporting goods store. If you don't want to spring for one, just try to fit lots of steps into your day in as many ways as possible.

Walk with a purpose. When you want to progress from baby steps to serious walking, set aside a 30-minute block of time each day for a fitness walk. This shouldn't be a stroll in the park. You should shoot for a speed of two miles in 30 minutes. A good way to gauge your time is to chart out a two-mile course in your car using the odometer. Or go to a local track.

The most important thing to remember is that you must burn more calories than you take in if you want to lose weight. And if you're just trying to maintain your weight, you need to burn at least an equal amount. But it takes effort, so whatever you do, expect to be tired afterward. Knowing that you're protecting your health by staying fit will make it all worthwhile.

Change dangerous flab to tight, flat abs

A "spare tire" around your waistline is a definite problem. Unwanted fat, especially at your midsection, increases your risk of heart disease, high blood pressure, diabetes, and some cancers. A recent study finds it can lead to lung problems as well.

Jump-start your workout with honey

Get more out of your workout with a surprising pick-me-up. A recent study of competitive bicyclists showed that honey gives you as big an energy jolt as glucose, the sugar used in sports gels and energy bars. Both honey and glucose boosted the bike riders' leg power and cut the time it took them to finish their race. Honey, though, has the added advantage of being much cheaper.

See for yourself if this natural sweetener gives you the energy to make it through a tougher workout. Before starting, wash down a tablespoon of honey with a cup of water. Any time you need an extra boost of energy during your workout, do the same.

Try it after you exercise, too. A post-workout spoonful appears to help your muscles recuperate. That's because honey is a great source of carbohydrates, and your body needs them to replace the ones you burned.

Naturally, you want to do something about it, but are gut-wrenching sit-ups the best way to get rid of a fat belly? Not according to Dr. Bryant Stamford, a professor of physiology at the University of Louisville, Kentucky. Writing in *The Physician And Sportsmedicine*, he points out there is no such thing as spot reduction. When you exercise, you don't necessarily burn fat from around the muscles you are using. If you want to get the most out of your abdominal workout, follow these tips.

Choose exercise that burns the most calories. The fat you burn when you exercise may come from anywhere on your body, so Stamford recommends doing the activities that use the most calories. He says you'd have to do hundreds of sit-ups to equal the calories you'd burn on a brisk walk or jog, for example.

Relax to stay trim. Exercise may be necessary for removing your potbelly, but reducing stress can help keep it off. For some reason, stress releases chemicals that cause fat to shift from other parts of your body to your waistline. Listening to music, talking things over with a friend or counselor, meditating, or doing yoga can help relieve stress. These practices also help you keep a positive attitude, which makes it easier to stick to your diet and exercise plan.

Tighten muscles for a sharper shape. Suck in your stomach when exercising, because a bouncing belly weakens the abdominal muscles. And don't forget to stretch your hamstrings. Strengthening these muscles on the back of your thighs helps prevent a swayback, which can make your stomach stick out even more.

Although they won't remove the fat, sit-ups can strengthen your abs, which protects your back as well. If full sit-ups seem too difficult, do just the second half, where you lower yourself down. Here's how:

- ⊷ Starting from a sitting position with hands at your sides, place your feet flat on the floor with your legs at a 90-degree angle. This way your abdominal muscles, not your legs and hips, will do the work.

- ⊷ Tense your belly and slowly — so your muscles work against gravity's downward pull — lower yourself until your back touches the floor.

- ⊷ Push yourself back up with your arms.

Repeat five times in the beginning, adding a few more each time you work out. To exercise your abdominal muscles a little harder, increase resistance by crossing your arms over your chest.

Drop pounds with a powerful potion

What would you say if someone offered you a tonic that could not only help you lose weight, but would improve your digestion, cushion your joints, keep your skin from drying out, and help your body heal after surgery? It's hard to say no to an offer like that, especially when it's safe, free, and flowing right into your kitchen.

Water, this natural fountain of youth, has zero calories, so substituting it for high-calorie beverages gives you a clear advantage. But don't think filling up on water will make you eat less at dinner. A Penn State University study found the popular practice of drinking a glass of water before meals to feel full doesn't reduce hunger.

A bowl of soup, however, just may do the trick. Not only does it work better than a glass of water, researchers found eating

Diuretics: Fast track to a heart attack

Taking diet pills may seem like a faster track to a slimmer figure than counting calories and exercising. But these medications can be dangerous, especially if you have heart problems, diabetes, or certain other diseases.

By the same token, don't be tempted to use diuretics, or water pills, to lose weight either. They can disturb your body's electrolyte balance and put you at risk of a heart attack. They are especially dangerous when combined with a low-protein diet, which can starve your heart muscle and disturb heart rhythms.

Using water pills when taking other medicines is also risky business. "People taking diuretics are particularly vulnerable to dehydration," says cardiologist Dr. David Calhoun, director of the University of Alabama Birmingham Hypertension Clinic.

"The combination of depleted fluid volume and medication," he warns, "can lead to problems such as dangerously low blood pressure, particularly for older patients who are sensitive to becoming dehydrated."

If you take medications, Calhoun says to be sure to drink at least the recommended six glasses of water each day — more when you exercise or spend a lot of time in the sun.

chicken and rice soup curbed the appetite better than eating chicken and rice casserole with the same ingredients plus drinking a glass of water.

Furthermore, it's the amount of food, the researchers say, not the number of calories it contains, that gives you a feeling of being full. So those with high water content satisfy the appetite just as much as the more calorie-dense foods. A large pasta salad made with carrots and zucchini, for example, fills you up better than a smaller portion of pasta without the veggies, but with an equal number of calories.

Fresh fruit in salads; lettuce, tomato, and sprouts on a turkey breast sandwich; and extra vegetables and beans in chili are other appetizing ways to fill up without adding lots of calories. But don't stop drinking water as well. It does far more than help you lose weight, and if you're like most people, you don't drink enough.

Startling secret to weight loss

A hidden cause of weight gain may make dropping 25 pounds as easy as giving up your favorite vegetables.

So says Rudy Rivera, M.D., who maintains food intolerances are to blame for many of the weight problems people suffer. In his book *Your Hidden Food Allergies Are Making You Fat*, co-authored by Roger D. Deutsch, he tells of his own struggle with being overweight. Once he identified his food culprits — among them, carrots, broccoli, and green beans — he says he finally slimmed down and felt healthy.

True food allergies cause immediate reactions such as hives or wheezing, and can be life-threatening. But when you're sensitive to a certain food, the reaction is not as obvious, Rivera says. It might not appear until hours or days later, and by then you wouldn't think of connecting it to something you ate. Even so, an allergic-type reaction is invading your body. Your white blood cells can swell and burst, irritating the other cells. The result? You may feel exhausted, have a migraine, or keep gaining weight.

Rivera believes a lot of obesity is linked to this food sensitivity cycle. He explains that after your body reacts to an offending food, it becomes low in serotonin — a feel-good chemical that has a calming effect on the brain. Because eating carbohydrates can raise serotonin levels, you find yourself craving things like sugary snacks. Even worse, you'll probably crave the very foods you're sensitive to.

But you can break the cycle by figuring out which foods your body can't process. You can try eliminating foods from your diet one at a time to see if you notice any improvement, but this can be difficult if you're sensitive to several foods. Rivera recommends the ALCAT test, a blood test for food intolerances. Along with identifying your problem foods, it tests for sensitivity to molds, chemicals such as preservatives, and food dyes. Rivera says once he stopped eating his trigger foods, he easily lost 25 pounds in a couple of months.

But you have to stay away from your problem foods for at least three months, he says. After that, you can eat small amounts of the food again, but only occasionally. To avoid reactions, you should rotate foods so you never eat any food more than once every four days, he notes.

Your insurance company should pay for the ALCAT test if your doctor orders it, but check first. Some experts believe these types of allergy tests are not effective. If your doctor won't order it, the company that designed the test can refer you to another doctor, or you can do it at home. For more information, go to the Web site <www.alcat.com> or contact: AMTL Corp., One Oakwood Blvd., Suite 130, Hollywood, FL 33020, 800-881-2685.

Trim the fat in Greek restaurants

Nutritionists have long touted the Mediterranean diet as a super meal plan that leads to a long and healthy life. But before you book nightly reservations at your local Greek restaurant, you should know the food they serve is not nearly as healthy as the food cooked in the old country. In fact, a recent survey shows it's loaded with heart-clogging, waist-thickening fat.

The true Greek diet consists of many fruits, vegetables, grains, and some olive oil. They only eat red meat a few times a month, and poultry and fish a few times a week. And saturated fat usually accounts for no more than 8 percent of calories. But in Greek restaurants, those healthy ideas have been turned upside down. Researchers found huge amounts of saturated fat in most of the main dishes, and much more meat than the Mediterranean diet calls for.

Nutrition experts say you should eat no more than 65 grams of fat a day, including less than 20 grams of saturated fat, for a 2,000-calorie-a-day diet. But even 20 grams of saturated fat is probably too much if you want to protect your arteries and heart. How can you eat Greek food and be heart healthy? Follow these guidelines to reap the benefits of a Mediterranean diet without the pitfalls.

Skip the sandwich. The average restaurant gyro — a pita bread sandwich filled with meat, raw vegetables, sometimes feta cheese, and a cucumber sauce — weighs in with 760 calories and 44 grams of total fat. Of those, nearly half are saturated — the kind of artery-blocking fat you should avoid like the plague. Don't be fooled into thinking this sandwich is traditional Mediterranean fare. The gyro hasn't been around very long, and anyone who eats these regularly probably won't be either.

Savor souvlaki. Happily, there are a few healthy choices on the menu. Souvlaki, which you may know as shish kebob, is a winner with its small amount of meat and hefty serving of vegetables on a skewer. An average serving of chicken souvlaki has only 260 calories with 8 grams of fat — only two of them saturated. The beef and lamb souvlaki are a bit higher on the fat scale but still within a healthy range.

Sideline the toppings. Even if you decide to play it safe and order a Greek salad, you're not out of the heart danger zone. Researchers found the average Greek salad has about 390 calories, 12 grams of saturated fat, and a total of 30 grams of fat. For a healthier salad, ask for the oil dressing and feta cheese on the side. That way, you can add just a tablespoon or two for flavor and keep from drowning in fat.

Split servings. Moussaka, a popular ground beef and eggplant casserole, chalks up a whopping 830 calories and 48 grams of fat. Again, roughly half the fat is saturated. Since Greek restaurants often serve huge portions, why not take advantage of that with a spouse or friend? Order one entrée and share it to cut 50 percent of the fat. Ask for extra vegetables as a side order. Or you can cut the meal in two when it arrives at your table, and eat only half of it. Ask for a to-go box, and warm up your leftovers for an enjoyable lunch the next day.

Splurge on dessert. The famous Greek dessert baklava, which is a flaky, honey and nut pastry, is not nearly as rich as many other desserts. A typical serving of baklava has 550 calories and 21 grams of fat, including five that are saturated. A lemon ice would be better, but baklava still beats apple pie with its 28 grams of fat, a fudge brownie sundae with 57 grams of fat, and the biggest dessert criminal — cheesecake — with 49 grams of fat, 31 of them saturated. Even so, researchers suggest you play it safe and share your baklava with a friend.

Stay super healthy with 50 top nutrition tips

- Put spinach on your sandwich instead of lettuce. A recent study found most people couldn't tell the difference, and spinach is much more nutritious.

- Eat your garnish. Restaurants often pretty up your plate with parsley or kale. Instead of admiring these nutritional powerhouses, eat them.

- Toss some blueberries in your morning cereal, muffin or pancake mix, or even in a bowl of ice cream.

- Instead of mayonnaise, butter, or cream cheese, try using mashed avocado as a spread.

- Use olive oil or canola oil instead of animal oils or other vegetable oils.

- Invest in a good set of nonstick cookware. You'll be able to use less fat when cooking.

- Use legumes (beans and peas) in soups and casseroles, and cut back on meat.

- Choose lean cuts of meat, and trim as much excess fat away as you can before cooking.

- Don't smother your baked potato with butter or sour cream. Instead, try topping it with salsa or even low-fat chili.

- Sauté vegetables in wine or broth instead of butter or oil.

- Add mashed avocado or pumpkin to mashed potatoes for a little extra nutrition. Use about one-fourth to one-half cup for every two cups of potatoes.

- Heat enhances the sweet taste of food, so if you serve sweet foods warm, you may be able to add less sugar.

- Yogurt "cheese" is a good substitute for sour cream. Line a strainer or funnel with cheesecloth or a paper coffee filter. Add plain yogurt and let it drain into a bowl overnight in the refrigerator. Simply discard the liquid, and you're ready to use the yogurt in your favorite recipe.

- If you chill soups and stews, most of the fat will solidify on top. Skim off the solid fat, and then heat and eat.

- Choose fruits and vegetables with the darkest colors to get the most vitamin C.

- Order your pizza with lots of veggies, and blot with a paper towel to absorb any excess grease.

- Add shredded apple to a peanut butter or grilled cheese sandwich.

- At your next cookout, add vegetables to the grill. Throw some asparagus spears on, or skewer chunks of onion, green pepper, tomatoes, and mushrooms.

- Grill a tropical kabob with chunks of pineapple, papaya, and ham.

- Bake a banana. Put a whole, ripe banana on a cookie sheet. Bake for 20 minutes at 350 degrees. Split the skin and sprinkle with nutmeg or cinnamon.

- Stuff bell peppers with cooked rice or pasta and tomato sauce. Cook in a muffin tin to help the peppers hold their shape.

- For salsa with a surprising sweet twist, mix chopped kiwifruit or papaya with tomatoes, green onions, and cilantro.

- Puree mangoes and use as a sauce for grilled chicken, pork, or fish.

- Make a yummy and attractive breakfast parfait. Layer low-fat yogurt, granola cereal, and fruit such as peaches, or pineapple in a parfait glass.

- Canned fruit is nutritious, but make sure you buy the kind packed in its own juice — not in calorie-laden syrup.

- Don't skip breakfast. If you're in a hurry, grab an apple, a bagel, or a banana.

- Bake your own bread, and add dried fruits, vegetables, or seeds for more taste and nutrition.

- Look for 100-percent fruit juice. Other fruit drinks usually contain more sugar than nutrition.

- Eat broth-based soups — they are far lower in fat than cream-based alternatives.

- Serve meat or poultry with cranberry sauce, salsa, or chutney, and skip the gravy.

- Don't let dining out become an excuse for pigging out. Most restaurants serve unnecessarily large portions. Split an entrée with someone else, or just eat half and ask for a doggie bag.

- Don't be fooled by fat-free foods. Many of them are still high in calories. Read labels carefully.

- When you just have to eat cake, try angel food cake topped with fresh fruit.

- Popcorn can be a high-fiber, low-calorie snack if you don't drench it in butter. If you don't like air-popped corn, try using a small amount of olive oil for a delicious healthy flavor.

- Nuts tend to be high in fat, but they also get high marks for nutrition, so include them in your diet. Just don't overdo it.

- Focus on your food. You'll eat less and enjoy your food more if you don't eat while working, watching television, or driving.

- Add brown or wild rice to casseroles and soups for more fiber and nutrition.

- Substitute mungbean paste for some of the butter in peanut butter cookies to lower fat and increase fiber.

- If you are bored with bananas but want the potassium, try something more exotic — like kiwifruit or mangoes.

- Microwave your vegetables to retain more of their vitamins and minerals.

- Toss steamed veggies with whole-wheat pasta to add more fiber to your diet.

- Grill fish by wrapping in foil with a little lemon juice and herbs.

- Blend up a fast, nutritious shake with low-fat milk, low-fat yogurt, ice cubes, and your favorite fruit.

- Bypass self-basting turkeys, which are injected with fat to make them moist. Baste your turkey with broth instead.

- Substitute unsweetened applesauce for up to half the butter or oil called for in your baking recipes.

- Sprinkle flaxseed on soups, salads, and hot or cold cereals.

- When dining out, always ask for sauces and salad dressings on the side, and then use them sparingly.

- Broil, bake, grill, steam, or poach meats and vegetables instead of frying or boiling them. You'll lower fat and retain nutrients.

↦ Replace the cream in your recipe with low-fat sour cream or low-fat evaporated milk.

↦ For more lycopene, choose sun-dried tomatoes over the fresh variety. Those packed in oil are best at helping your body absorb this cancer-fighting nutrient.

Folk Remedy

Japanese women have kept a secret about weight loss for centuries. But now the cat's out of the bag — or teacup. Drinking three to five cups of green tea at each meal helps boost your metabolism, which means you burn calories faster. In addition, green tea helps you lose extra water weight.

WOUNDS AND INJURIES

Folk remedies manage minor emergencies

When you're traveling, you never know what's going to hit you. Whether it's a bout of heartburn, a cold during ski season, or a sunburn at the beach, there's no substitute for being prepared.

You could buy a prepackaged first-aid kit off the shelf of your local pharmacy, but if you assemble your own, you can combine safe commercial medications with folk remedies — all at a low cost.

Here are some old-fashioned cures that are easy to take with you.

- **Baking soda.** A little box of this miracle powder can do a lot. For starters, mix one-half teaspoon with one-half cup of water and drink it down for quick indigestion relief.

> ### What is it?
> A wound is defined as any break in the soft tissues of your body — for example a bite, cut, puncture, or tear. Injuries are more general — almost any kind of damage or trauma to your body. They can range from a skinned knee to a concussion. Most injuries are an everyday thing and need only a good cleaning and a bandage. Sometimes, though, they're more than skin deep and call for medical attention.
>
> Symptoms:
> - Bleeding
> - Pain
> - Swelling and redness
> - Break or tear in skin
> - Shock (paleness, rapid breathing, blank expression)

✧ **Banana peel or potato slice.** When you can't find an ordinary bandage, these will take the "ouch" out of a nick or scrape. Just place the inside of a banana peel over your scratch, or tape a thin slice of raw potato to it.

✧ **Echinacea.** Whether as a tea or supplement, this herb is your cold's worst enemy. It will ease the sniffling, sneezing, and achiness of wintertime woes in no time at all.

✧ **Ginger.** For centuries, sailors have relied on ginger to keep them free of seasickness. For easy storage in your first-aid kit, try candied or crystallized ginger. An hour before you go on board, eat two chunks — each about one inch square by one-quarter inch thick. Then have one or two more every four hours as needed.

✧ **Panty hose and oats.** To ease the itchiness of poison ivy, sunburn, or some other rash, cut off the foot of an old pair of panty hose. Fill it with rolled oats, tie the end, and hold the sack under the running faucet in your tub. Then settle down for a deep soak.

✧ **Rice and a sock.** Fill an old sock with uncooked rice or birdseed and then sew it tightly shut. Either keep it in the freezer for a cold compress, or toss it in the microwave for hot relief. Make sure to place a cup of water in the microwave with it so the sock doesn't overheat and catch fire. This is great for sore muscles, migraines, or aching joints.

✧ **Rubbing alcohol.** Fill a resealable plastic freezer bag with a mixture of water and rubbing alcohol and throw it in the freezer. For a softer, less frozen ice pack, add more alcohol.

✧ **Salt.** Stir up one-fourth teaspoon of salt and one-half cup of warm water. Gargle and — presto — no more sore throat. Also, unstuff your stuffy nose, with a homemade saline nasal spray. Mix one-half teaspoon salt with eight ounces of warm water. Use either an empty nasal spray bottle or a bulb syringe.

↬ **Superglue.** For faster healing of a paper cut or dry, cracked skin, drop on a bit of superglue. Just don't try this remedy on deep or bleeding cuts, and let the glue dry thoroughly before touching anything — especially your eyes.

↬ **Take-out condiments.** A big ice pack won't work for tiny injuries. Instead, save up the individual packets of mustard and ketchup you can get at any fast-food joint. Keep them in the freezer, and they'll come in handy for little hurts.

↬ **Tea bags.** If the sun left you well done, try dropping two or three tea bags into your bath. Or use moist gauze to hold them directly onto your burns.

↬ **Vinegar.** For immediate relief from a sting or bite, dab vinegar on with a cotton ball.

↬ **Vitamin C.** As soon as a nasty bug stings you, pop 1,000 to 1,500 milligrams of this wonder vitamin. It will act like a natural antihistamine to help soothe the sting and swelling.

↬ **White glue or tape.** Lift out a splinter painlessly. Just dab on some white glue, let it dry, then peel the glue and the splinter right off. A piece of tape will work well on those tiny splinters you can't see.

Remember that pain, swelling, and other symptoms are your body's way of saying something is wrong. Pay attention and you'll recognize which everyday ailments and accidents you can treat yourself and which require professional help. Ear pain, toothaches, and vomiting, for instance, are more likely to need a doctor's call.

Interest-free relief for jellyfish stings

Don't go to the beach without your credit card — not for financial emergencies, but for jellyfish emergencies.

Simply whip out your card if one of these floating creatures stings you, then gently scrape it over the affected area to remove any stingers left in your skin. The edge of a knife blade works, too.

Pack on the ice for the pain and swelling. If it's a serious sting, try diluted vinegar. Just never flush a sting with fresh water, since this can actually make it worse.

You may have heard credit cards are handy for bee stings, too, but they aren't necessarily the best remedy. Since the stinger can pump you full of venom in 20 seconds or less, the key is getting it out as quickly as possible. So, it doesn't matter how you do it just as long as it's fast. Even pulling it out by hand works. Experts say don't worry — you won't squeeze more venom into your bloodstream.

If you can't remember the last time you got a tetanus shot, even a minor cut or wound could require medical attention. Better yet, prevent tetanus by getting a booster every ten years.

Bargain ways to beat bug bites

Don't spend a fortune on sprays and creams to soothe bug bites and stings. And don't expose yourself and your loved ones to harsh chemical bug repellents either. You can find a virtual pharmacy of natural alternatives at home — folk remedies that are tried-and-true ways to get quick relief.

Repel bugs naturally. The best way to relieve bug bites is to avoid them in the first place. A simple — and free — way to ward off mosquitoes, yellow jackets, and the like is to keep a few things in mind when you get dressed. Avoid wearing perfume or cologne, and leave your shiny jewelry indoors. These, along with bright colors and flowery-print clothing, attract bugs. Nature also provides it's own collection of bug fighters, which work just as well as any store-bought repellent. You can find all of these fresh herbs and oils at your local grocer or health food store.

- ⊷ **Lavender.** An essential oil made from this plant is great for warding off gnats and mosquitoes. Just mix two parts lavender oil with one part rubbing alcohol.

- ⊷ **Parsley, lemon balm, or basil.** Rub the fresh leaves of any of these herbs on your skin if you want to stay welt-free.

- ⊷ **Garlic juice.** People on the island of Sardinia douse themselves with this potent solution to keep away those dreaded bloodsuckers — mosquitoes, of course.

- ⊷ **Thyme.** Ancient Greeks burned thyme to discourage stinging pests. Dried thyme will keep bugs out of your linen closet, too.

Find natural relief. If a creepy crawly still gets you, don't fret. Just try one of these homespun wonders. They might do away with the itch and irritation of a bite or sting.

- ⊷ **Aspirin.** To swat the discomfort of bug bites, you don't have to swallow this over-the-counter drug. Put the aspirin right on your welt. First, make sure the stinger isn't still in your skin. (If it is, pull it out or scrape it away with a credit card or knife.) Then, just crush an aspirin tablet, wet it slightly, and bandage it over the sting. You can also use other nonsteroidal anti-inflammatories (NSAIDs), like ibuprofen. For even more relief, try dousing your bites with an antihistamine. Just make sure you're not allergic.

- ⊷ **Basil.** This herb is good for something besides topping tomatoes and mozzarella cheese. Crush fresh basil leaves and rub them on your bug bite for some sweet relief. You can keep the basil in place with a loose bandage.

- **Onions.** Stop crying over that itching and swelling. Mash a fresh slice of onion and apply it, juices and all, to your sting. Onions contain phytochemicals, natural substances that will help reduce your swelling and pain.

- **Hot peppers.** Just like an onion, these fiery remedies work wonders when you crush them and spread over your sting. A hot pepper won't lower the inflammation of a bug bite, but it will heat up your skin enough to take your mind off it. A few drops of hot sauce will do the trick, too. If your skin becomes too irritated, rinse the area immediately.

- **Peppermint and witch hazel.** Peppermint oil can irritate your skin, so, like a hot pepper, a dab will make you forget your itchy bites. Witch hazel, on the other hand, can soothe and reduce swelling. That's why they make a perfect pair. Just mix two drops of peppermint essential oil for every ounce of witch hazel. Keep this precious potion in a cool, dark spot, and use a cotton ball to dab on as needed.

- **Baking soda and rubbing alcohol.** Mix these two common household ingredients into a paste for some quick and easy relief.

Test a small amount of any home remedy on the inside of your forearm, especially if you have allergies or sensitive skin. Don't use it if you develop redness or itching within 24 hours.

Kitchen remedies that can save your skin

When life's little mishaps lead to minor cuts and scrapes, head for your kitchen. Many everyday items in your refrigerator or cupboard are natural remedies that work just as well as medicines from the pharmacy.

Papaya. This tropical fruit is a traditional therapy in the Caribbean and Africa, and now modern science praises it, too. A dressing of mashed, unripe papaya removes dead tissue, encourages new skin growth, and reduces infection. It's particularly effective on skin ulcers and burns.

If you want to try this remedy, spread a new layer evenly and thickly over your wound every day. Be warned though, papaya can burn when you first put it on.

Honey. Scientists are buzzing with news about honey's miraculous healing powers. This sweet treat can keep your wound clean, kill bacteria, prevent scarring, and help your body heal itself. Even your average supermarket honey bear can spread some healing, but unprocessed honeys — like you find at natural foods stores — work better. If you want the very best, try Active Manuka Honey. It comes from New Zealand and is available over the Internet. Whatever type of honey you use, apply one ounce of it for every four square inches of wound. It's best to spread the honey onto a bandage rather than directly onto your skin.

Cinnamon. Believe it or not, this spice is a complete healing package that can numb your pain, kill infection-causing bacteria, and stop bleeding. After you wash and dry your cut, shake on some cinnamon powder and cover with a bandage.

Before you treat any wound at home, make sure it's not serious enough to need professional care. If your injury is minor, clean it by gently rinsing under running water or saline. Then — relax. When your body is trying to heal itself, stress is the last thing you need. Research shows stress weakens your immune system and slows down healing time.

Simple solution for icing injuries

You know that icing a sprain, twist, bang, or other injury is a key step in good first aid. Ice lowers swelling and numbs the pain. But icing the old-fashioned way means sitting around and holding an ice pack to your injury. Let plastic wrap do all that bothersome holding for you.

Just cut a roll of plastic wrap in half. Then take one side of it and use as much as it takes to secure the ice pack over your injury. The ice will stay in place while you're free to move around. You can even use plastic wrap to strap ice onto your back if that's where the pain is.

Don't let an injury keep you down. With this simple solution, you can stay moderately active while helping yourself heal.

How to keep good makeup from going bad

People do some dangerous things for the sake of beauty. Thousands of years ago, Egyptians lined their eyes with malachite, lead, or soot. Not only was this dramatic look uncomfortable, but unsafe, as well. Then, for years, women lost their hair from bleaches made with lye, and actually died from lead poisoning as they powdered their skin with white lead. You'd think the time of fashion gone wrong would be past. But in the United States, manufacturers don't need Food and Drug Administration (FDA) approval before they sell cosmetics, and the government doesn't regulate cosmetic expiration dates. Unbelievably, manufacturers are encouraged to set their own safety guidelines.

Wealthy Egyptian women were often buried with cosmetics so they could use them in the afterlife. But you certainly don't want to wear the same cosmetics for all eternity. Follow these tips to keep your good looks and good health.

366

Replace mascara often. Eye makeup is especially dangerous to keep for a long time. You can develop serious eye infections from old or contaminated products — even run the risk of blindness. Never mind how little you used, or how much you paid for it. To protect yourself from infection, buy new mascara every three months. And if it dries out, never add water or saliva. That's a sure way to start a bacteria colony. If you do get an eye infection, stop wearing eye makeup immediately, and throw out any cosmetics that might have touched your eye. And, of course, see your doctor.

Don't share makeup. Forget what you learned in kindergarten about sharing. When it comes to cosmetics, it's best to be selfish. Otherwise, you could end up swapping bacteria. Never use "testers" at cosmetic counters, either — this is just large-scale sharing. An FDA study of these shared cosmetics was a real eye-opener. They found fungi in more than 10 percent of the products tested. Frighteningly, the worst offender was eye makeup.

Question "natural" labeling. Cosmetics labeled "all natural" seem like a healthy choice. But what exactly does natural mean? After all, bacteria are natural, but certainly not good for your skin.

Egg-cellent treatment for a sty

You don't need a hard-boiled detective to track down a simple home remedy for eye disorders. All you need is a hard-boiled egg.

If you have a sty or a cyst on your eye, your doctor might tell you to apply a hot compress for 10 minutes three or four times a day. With its oval shape, an egg makes a perfect compress for your eye.

Just hard-boil an egg, let it cool until it's warm (not scalding hot) or wrap it in a washcloth and place it on the infected eye for 10 minutes. When it's time for your next 10-minute session, simply re-heat the same egg.

Although the industry doesn't have strict guidelines for natural products, usually, you can count on the ingredients coming directly from plants or animals, and not made in a lab. However, even plants can be contaminated with pesticides and fertilizers. In addition, natural cosmetics tend to become contaminated faster since they don't contain laboratory-made preservatives.

Store products properly. To slow down contamination, keep your cosmetics away from heat and sunlight and always put the lid back on tightly.

Last of all, use common sense. Apply makeup with clean hands to a clean face. And if any of your makeup looks or smells funny, throw it away. Despite all the pressure to be beautiful, your health is still more important than your looks.

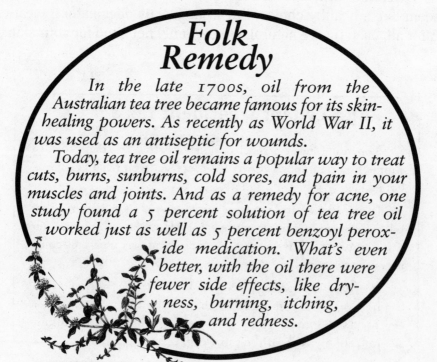

Folk
Remedy

In the late 1700s, oil from the Australian tea tree became famous for its skin-healing powers. As recently as World War II, it was used as an antiseptic for wounds.

Today, tea tree oil remains a popular way to treat cuts, burns, sunburns, cold sores, and pain in your muscles and joints. And as a remedy for acne, one study found a 5 percent solution of tea tree oil worked just as well as 5 percent benzoyl peroxide medication. What's even better, with the oil there were fewer side effects, like dryness, burning, itching, and redness.

WRINKLES

Straighten out your diet to prevent wrinkles

Going to the grocery store for a face lift? Not exactly. But you will find its shelves stocked with items that can either fast forward or turn back time.

Your skin is your body's largest organ, and so it's a huge target for free radicals. These unstable molecules form as you process oxygen. They travel throughout your body, damaging cells and causing all sorts of havoc — including wrinkles. You can't help producing free radicals, but you can help neutralize them.

Eat smart for smoother skin. Certain foods can actually protect your face from wrinkles, according to Australian researcher, Dr. Mark L. Wahlqvist of Monash University in Melbourne. He found that if foods contain powerful antioxidants — whether in the form of vitamins, carotenoids, polyphenols, or other phytochemicals — they counteract dangerous free radicals.

What is it?

As you age, your body naturally produces less collagen and elastin — connective tissues that make your skin firm and supple. The layer of fat under your skin also begins to disappear. As a result, the skin, especially on your face, starts to sag and wrinkle.

Your genes, in general, determine when this occurs and how fast it progresses. But smoking and too much exposure to the sun can speed up the process.

Symptoms:
- Sagging
- Lines, ridges, creases, and furrows
- Dryness

Wahlqvist and his team of researchers learned these foods seem to fight wrinkles:

Eggs	Cherries
Yogurt	Grapes
Spinach	Melons
Eggplant	Prunes
Asparagus	Dried fruit
Celery	Apples
Garlic	Pears
Onions	Multigrain bread
Nuts	Jam
Lima beans	Tea
Olives	Water

In addition, foods like olive oil contain monounsaturated fat, which resists skin cell damage.

It's easy to fit these into your weekly menu, and with so many to choose from, you can still enjoy a wide variety of dishes. Meals that blend vegetables, legumes, and olive oil — like those in a typical Greek diet — offer even more protection against wrinkles.

Avoid wrinkle-causing foods. Amid all the good news, researchers also discovered that certain foods have the opposite effect — they seem to encourage wrinkling. Saturated fat does not protect against sun damage and sugary products actually deteriorate your overall skin health.

Milk (full-fat)	Butter
Margarine	Ice cream
Red meat	Potatoes
Soft drinks	Cakes, pastries, etc.

Try to eliminate or cut back on these foods. Swap skim or fat-free milk for whole milk, water for soft drinks, fish for beef or pork, and fruit for sweet, sugary desserts. This just might be the recipe for a younger-looking you.

Worry less about wrinkles

If your face shows your age all too clearly, a new wrinkle in cancer research could mean good news for you. Doctors in England speculate that if you have wrinkles, you might actually be protected from skin cancer.

Most people believe that wrinkling indicates sun damage and a higher risk of skin cancer. But, that's not the whole story. According to Dr. Christopher E.M. Griffiths, professor of dermatology at the University of Manchester's Hope Hospital, there are different types of skin and they react differently to sun exposure.

Ultraviolet rays from the sun destroy the elastic collagen fibers in all types of skin. If you are wrinkled, that means your skin type repairs itself but doesn't replace the collagen. If you have smooth skin, on the other hand, your skin is replacing the damaged collagen.

Griffith believes this amount of collagen in your skin could affect your risk of skin cancer in a roundabout way. A substance called transforming growth factor (TGF)-beta helps rebuild the collagen. However, it also suppresses your immune system — and a weakened immune system has more trouble fighting off cancer. In other words, the same process that keeps your skin smooth and firm might also allow cancer to develop. "This is speculative!" stresses Griffiths.

He first noticed that his patients with basal cell carcinoma, the most common form of skin cancer, had fewer wrinkles than other patients. Then, a study of over 200 people shed further light. Those with heavily wrinkled faces were up to 90 percent less likely to develop basal cell carcinoma than smooth-skinned people.

Unfortunately, you can't control the type of skin you have. So, it is still important you take the usual steps to protect yourself from the sun. "It's best to avoid sunbathing and use high factor sunscreens," Griffiths says.

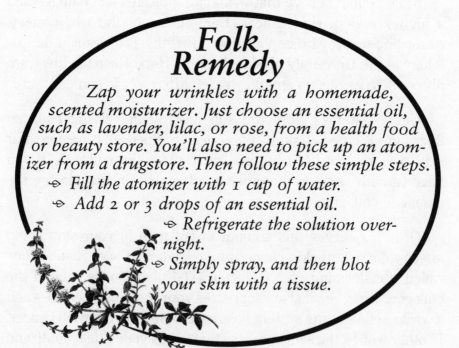

Folk Remedy

Zap your wrinkles with a homemade, scented moisturizer. Just choose an essential oil, such as lavender, lilac, or rose, from a health food or beauty store. You'll also need to pick up an atomizer from a drugstore. Then follow these simple steps.

⁍ *Fill the atomizer with 1 cup of water.*
⁍ *Add 2 or 3 drops of an essential oil.*
⁍ *Refrigerate the solution overnight.*
⁍ *Simply spray, and then blot your skin with a tissue.*

INDEX

Bacteria *(continued)*
  rheumatoid
    arthritis and 290
  shellfish and 127
  tooth decay and 322
  Vibrio vulnificus 128
  vinegar for 127
Baking soda
  for bug bites 364
  for diarrhea 112
  for indigestion 359
  for skin rash 12
Baldness, prostate
    cancer and 280
Basil, for bug
    bites 363
Beans, for high
    cholesterol 156
Beta carotene, *see also*
    Vitamin A
  for memory loss 225
  for oral cancer 312
  for prostate cancer
    278
  sources of 54, 225
Bilberries, for
    vision 119
Biofeedback
  for migraines 144
  for tinnitus 316
Black cohosh, for
    menopause 234
Bladder control, *see*
    Urinary
    incontinence
Bleeding, aspirin
    and 159
Blood pressure, *see*
    High blood pressure
Body language 82
Body Mass Index
    (BMI) 343
Bone density, breast
    cancer and 52
Botox 141
BPH (benign prostatic
    hyperplasia) 281
Brain tumor 145
Breakfast, for memory
    loss 227

Breast cancer 44-53
Bromelain
  for diarrhea 111
  for rheumatoid
    arthritis 293
Bruxism 323
Bug bites, natural
    remedies for 362
Butcher's broom, for
    varicose veins 335

C

Caffeine
  chronic pain and 245
  for asthma 38
  panic attacks and 29
  tinnitus and 317
Calcium
  constipation and 74
  dangers of 273
  for Alzheimer's
    disease 17
  for gingivitis 136
  for menopause 236
  for migraines 143
  for muscle cramps
    247
  for osteoporosis 266
  non-dairy sources
    of 224
  sources of 266
  supplements 271
Calendula, for skin
    rash 10
Cancer, *see* Breast
    cancer, Prostate
    cancer *and* Skin
    cancer
Capsaicin, for
    psoriasis 285
Carotenoids, *see*
    Beta carotene
Cascara sagrada, for
    constipation 71
Castor oil, for

constipation 71
Cataracts 54-57
Celery, for high blood
    pressure 180
Cereal, for
    constipation 72
Chamomile
  for anxiety 30
  for skin rash 10
Cheese, heart disease
    and 157
Chewing gum, for
    heartburn 151
Chicken soup, for
    colds 66
Chocolate
  heartburn and 148
  toothache and 324
  urinary incontinence
    and 328
Cholesterol, *see* High
    cholesterol
Chondroitin, for
    osteoarthritis 258
Cinnamon
  for diabetes 107
  for wounds 365
Cloves, for
    toothache 325
Coal tar, for
    psoriasis 285
Coffee, *see also*
    Caffeine
  for depression 89
  for kidney stones
    220
  for low blood
    pressure 175
  high blood pressure
    and 174
  rheumatoid arthritis
    and 290
  urinary incontinence
    and 328
Cold and flu 58-66
Colon cancer
  fiber and 68
Computers, eyestrain
    and 117

Concussion 145
Constipation 67-75
  varicose veins
  and 331
Copper, for rheumatoid
  arthritis 302
Corticosteroids, high
  blood pressure
  and 176
Counseling, for
  anxiety 28
Cramp bark, for
  muscle pain 243
Cranberry juice, for
  urinary incontinence
  330
Credit card, for
  jellyfish stings 362
Cucumber, for puffy
  eyes 210
Cyclosporine, high
  blood pressure
  and 176

D

Dandruff 288
DASH diet 167
Daylight savings
  time 204
Dementia, *see*
  Alzheimer's disease
Dental problems, *see*
  Gingivitis *and*
  Toothache
Dentures 322
Depression 76-89
  migraines and 138
  stroke and 202
Dermatitis, atopic 11
Diabetes 90-98,
  100-107
  gingivitis and 133
Diarrhea 108-113
Dieting, *see* Weight
  problems
Diuretics 349

Driving, eyestrain
  and 117
Drug-herb
  interactions 88, 299
Drugs, *see* Medication
Dysphagia 201

E

E. coli
  (Escherichia coli)
  diarrhea and 111
  foods for 123
  garlic for 65
  petting zoos and 123
  produce and 125
Earplugs, for
  tinnitus 319
Echinacea, for colds
  59, 360
Eczema 11
Eggs
  for puffy eyes 210
  for sty 367
  heart disease and
  157
  substitutes for 189
Environmental
  Protection Agency
  (EPA) 130
Erectile dysfunction,
  see Impotence
Estrogen
  breast cancer and 53
  for high blood
  pressure 231
  for memory loss 231
  for osteoporosis 267
  urinary
  incontinence
  and 326
Estrogen replacement
  therapy (ERT)
  for Alzheimer's
  disease 19
  for osteoarthritis

231
Eucalyptus oil, for
  headaches 146
Evening primrose oil,
  for rheumatoid
  arthritis 296
Exercise
  asthma and 38
  for Alzheimer's
  disease 20
  for breast cancer 48
  for colds and flu 58
  for constipation 68
  for depression 78
  for diabetes 91, 94
  for high blood
  pressure 168
  for muscle pain 239
  for osteoarthritis 252
  for osteoporosis 268
  for rheumatoid
  arthritis 291
  for stroke 195
  for tinnitus 316
  for varicose veins
  331
  rosacea and 305
  weight loss and 344
Eyestrain 114-119

F

Falls 21-23
  urinary incontinence
  and 330
Fast food, asthma
  and 36
Fat, *see also*
  Monounsaturated,
  Polyunsaturated
  and Saturated fats
  Alzheimer's disease
  and 16
  breast cancer and
  51
  cataracts and 56

G

Reflux, *see* Heartburn
Relationships, for high
blood pressure 177
Rheumatoid arthritis
(RA) 289-301
Riboflavin
for migraines 143
sources of 143
Roller coasters, stroke
and 199
Rosacea 303-307
Rosemary, for
memory loss 229
Rubbing alcohol
for bug bites 364
for injuries 360

S

Salad bars, food
poisoning and 122
Salicylates 255
Salmonella
garlic for 65
produce and 125
Salt
cataracts and 55
for headaches 138
for sore throat 360
high blood pressure
and 170
osteoporosis and 267
sources of 172
SAM-e (S-adenosyl-
methionine) 31
Saturated fat
high cholesterol
and 182
wrinkles and 370
Saw palmetto, for
BPH 281
Scleritis 300
Seasonal Affective
Disorder (SAD) 83
Selenium
for colds and flu 58
for depression 77

for prostate
cancer 278
sources of 77
Senna, for
constipation 71
Serotonin syndrome 88
Serotonin, heartburn
and 148
Sexual difficulties
205, 235, *see also*
Impotence
Shellfish, food
poisoning and 127
Sinusitis 145, 323
Sit-ups 348
Sjogren's syndrome
299
Skin cancer 308-312
wrinkles and 371
Skin problems, *see*
Allergy, Psoriasis,
Rosacea, *and* Skin
cancer
Skin rash
jewelry and 8
natural remedies
for 9
toiletries and 7
Sleep
for anxiety 26
for memory loss 227
heartburn and 148
kidney stones
and 218
Sleep apnea 207
menopause and 231
Sleep deprivation
dangers of 204
depression and 79
irritable bowel
syndrome and 213
Smoking
cataracts and 56
flying and 162
gingivitis and 133
irritability and 164
memory loss and 227
rheumatoid
arthritis and 289

stroke and 194
Snoring 207
Soda
memory loss and 18
weight loss and 340
Soy milk 274
Soy, menopause
and 236
Spices, rosacea
and 307
Spirituality, for
rheumatoid
arthritis 291
Splinters 361
St. John's wort
cataracts and 57
depression and 86
drug interactions
with 88
for menopause 234
Statins, for Alzheimer's
disease 18
Stinging nettle, for
BPH 282
Stress, *see also*
Anxiety
breast cancer and 47
colds and 62
diabetes and 106
flu shots and 61
forgiveness for 63
gingivitis and 135
health problems
and 25
irritable bowel
syndrome and 213
psoriasis and 284
rosacea and 305
tinnitus and 314
weight loss and 347
Stretching, for muscle
pain 239
Stroke 194-203
aspirin and 159
Sty 367
Sugar
gingivitis and 135
irritable bowel
syndrome and 212